Chapter 1: Fertility

Chapter 2: Reproductive ethics

Introduction

REPRODUCTION & FERTILITY is Volume 319 in the **ISSUES** series. The aim of the series is to offer current, diverse information about important issues in our world, from a UK perspective.

ABOUT TITLE

Fertility is often taken for granted by young people, but this book examines the facts surrounding the issue. It separates myth from fact, looks at medical conditions that can affect fertility and considers the complex feelings surrounding the struggle to conceive. It also looks at fertility treatments, such as IVF, and the controversy surrounding topics like three-parent babies, mitochondrial donation and sex-selection.

OUR SOURCES

Titles in the **ISSUES** series are designed to function as educational resource books, providing a balanced overview of a specific subject.

The information in our books is comprised of facts, articles and opinions from many different sources, including:

⇨ Newspaper reports and opinion pieces

⇨ Website factsheets

⇨ Magazine and journal articles

⇨ Statistics and surveys

⇨ Government reports

⇨ Literature from special interest groups.

A NOTE ON CRITICAL EVALUATION

Because the information reprinted here is from a number of different sources, readers should bear in mind the origin of the text and whether the source is likely to have a particular bias when presenting information (or when conducting their research). It is hoped that, as you read about the many aspects of the issues explored in this book, you will critically evaluate the information presented.

It is important that you decide whether you are being presented with facts or opinions. Does the writer give a biased or unbiased report? If an opinion is being expressed, do you agree with the writer? Is there potential bias to the 'facts' or statistics behind an article?

ASSIGNMENTS

In the back of this book, you will find a selection of assignments designed to help you engage with the articles you have been reading and to explore your own opinions. Some tasks will take longer than others and there is a mixture of design, writing and research-based activities that you can complete alone or in a group.

Useful weblinks

www.belfasttelegraph.co.uk

www.bionews.org.uk

www.bma.org.uk

www.bounty.com

www.breastcancercare.org.uk

www.bupa.co.uk

www.care.org.uk

www.theconversation.com

www.counselling-directory.org.uk

www.createhealth.org

www.thefword.org.uk

GOV.UK

www.theguardian.com

www.hfea.gov.uk

www.huffingtonpost.co.uk

www.ibtimes.co.uk

www.miscarriageassociation.org.uk

www.nhs.uk

www.rcog.org.uk

www.surrogacyuk.org

www.wellcome.ac.uk

www.yougov.co.uk

FURTHER RESEARCH

At the end of each article we have listed its source and a website that you can visit if you would like to conduct your own research. Please remember to critically evaluate any sources that you consult and consider whether the information you are viewing is accurate and unbiased.

Reproduction & Fertility

Series Editor: Cara Acred

Volume 319

Independence Educational Publishers

First published by Independence Educational Publishers

The Studio, High Green

Great Shelford

Cambridge CB22 5EG

England

© Independence 2017

ISBN-13: 978 1 86168 769 2

Printed in Great Britain

Zenith Print Group

Fertility: the facts

Conception is when a woman's egg is fertilised by a man's sperm, and then implants itself into the woman's womb. Most couples don't have a problem getting pregnant.

For most couples, regular unprotected sex is all it takes to conceive a child.

If you're trying for a baby or thinking of doing so in the future, knowing the basic facts about fertility can be helpful.

The monthly cycle

Every month, hormonal changes in a woman's body cause the ovaries to release a single egg. This egg passes into the fallopian tubes, which link the ovaries to the uterus (womb).

At the same time, the lining of the womb thickens. This is to prepare it for the possibility of receiving a fertilised egg.

If fertilisation does not occur, the womb lining will break down and will be shed through the vagina. This is a woman's period. The period is made up of the womb lining and a small amount of blood.

Women of childbearing age have a period approximately every 28 days, although the length of the cycle can vary and between 24 and 35 days is common.

If a woman has unprotected sex with a man around the time of her egg being released, sperm from her partner may fertilise her egg while it is in the fallopian tube. The fertilised egg will then travel to the womb and become embedded in its lining, where it will start to grow.

How conception happens

An egg can be fertilised by sperm during the 12 to 24 hours after it has been released from the ovaries.

Sperm can survive in the fallopian tubes for up to seven days, so fertilisation can occur even if sperm entered the fallopian tubes before an egg was released.

During conception, a single sperm from a man penetrates the egg of a woman. The sperm carries the father's genes, while the mother's genes are contained in the egg. Once the egg has been fertilised by a single sperm, no more sperm can enter.

The fertilised egg, called a zygote, continues to move down the fallopian tubes, until it reaches the womb. Here, it will implant itself into the lining of the womb (about six to ten days after ovulation), where it begins to grow.

Until eight weeks after conception, the implanted zygote is called an embryo. After this it is called a foetus.

For most women, the first sign that they are pregnant is a missed period. A few days after that missed period, a urine test can confirm the pregnancy.

Urine tests for pregnancy are available through your GP or family planning clinic. You can buy a test to do at home at your local pharmacy or supermarket.

3 October 2014

⇨ The above information is reprinted with kind permission from NHS Choices. Please visit www.nhs.uk for further information.

© NHS Choices 2016

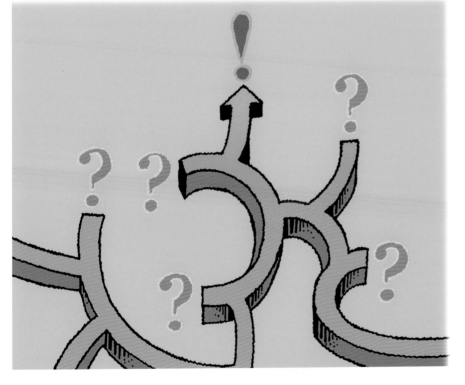

Infertility

Infertility is when a couple can't get pregnant (conceive), despite having regular unprotected sex.

Around one in seven couples may have difficulty conceiving. This is approximately 3.5 million people in the UK.

About 84% of couples will conceive naturally within one year if they have regular unprotected sex (every two or three days).

For couples who've been trying to conceive for more than three years without success, the likelihood of getting pregnant naturally within the next year is 25% or less.

Some women get pregnant quickly, but for others it can take longer. It's a good idea to see your GP if you haven't conceived after one year of trying.

Women aged 36 and over, and anyone who's already aware they may have fertility problems, should see their GP sooner. Your GP can check for common causes of fertility problems and suggest treatments that could help.

Infertility is only usually diagnosed when a couple haven't managed to conceive after one year of trying.

There are two types of infertility:

⇨ **primary infertility** – where someone who's never conceived a child in the past has difficulty conceiving

⇨ **secondary infertility** – where someone has had one or more pregnancies in the past, but is having difficulty conceiving again.

Treating infertility

Fertility treatments include:

⇨ **medical treatment** – for lack of regular ovulation

⇨ **surgical procedures** – such as treatment for endometriosis, repair of the fallopian tubes, or removal of scarring (adhesions) within the womb or abdominal cavity

⇨ **assisted conception** – this may be intrauterine insemination (IUI) or in-vitro fertilisation (IVF).

The treatment offered will depend on what's causing your fertility problems and what's available from your local clinical commissioning group (CCG).

Private treatment is also available, but it can be expensive and there's no guarantee it will be successful.

It's important to choose a private clinic carefully. You can ask your GP for advice, and should make sure you choose a clinic that's licensed by the Human Fertilisation and Embryology Authority (HFEA).

Some treatments for infertility, such as IVF, can cause complications.

For example:

⇨ **multiple pregnancy** – if more than one embryo is placed in the womb as part of IVF treatment, there's an increased chance of having twins; this may not seem like a bad thing, but it significantly increases the risk of complications for you and your babies

⇨ **ectopic pregnancy** – the risk of having an ectopic pregnancy is slightly increased if you have IVF.

What causes infertility?

There are many possible causes of infertility, and fertility problems can affect either the man or the woman. However, in a quarter of cases it isn't possible to identify the cause.

In women, common causes of infertility include:

⇨ lack of regular ovulation, the monthly release of an egg

⇨ blocked or damaged fallopian tubes

⇨ endometriosis – where tissue that behaves like the lining of the womb (the endometrium) is found outside the womb.

In men, the most common cause of infertility is poor-quality semen.

Risk factors

There are also a number of factors that can affect fertility in both men and women.

These include:

⇨ **age** – female fertility and, to a lesser extent, male fertility decline with age; in women, the biggest decrease in fertility begins during the mid-30s

⇨ **weight** – being overweight or obese (having a body mass index (BMI) of 30 or over) reduces fertility; in women, being overweight or severely underweight can affect ovulation

⇨ **sexually transmitted infections (STIs)** – several STIs, including chlamydia, can affect fertility

⇨ **smoking** – can affect fertility in both sexes: smoking (including passive smoking) affects a woman's chance of conceiving, while in men there's an association between smoking and reduced semen quality

⇨ **alcohol** – for women planning to get pregnant, the safest approach is not to drink alcohol at all to keep risks to your baby to a minimum; for men, drinking too much alcohol can affect the quality of sperm (the chief medical officers for the UK recommend men and women should drink no more than 14 units of alcohol a week, which should be spread evenly over three days or more)

⇨ **environmental factors** – exposure to certain pesticides, solvents and metals has been shown to affect fertility, particularly in men

⇨ **stress** – can affect your relationship with your partner and cause a loss of sex drive; in severe cases, stress may also affect ovulation and sperm production.

There's no evidence to suggest caffeinated drinks, such as tea, coffee and colas, are associated with fertility problems.

14 February 2017

⇨ The above information is reprinted with kind permission from NHS Choices. Please visit www.nhs.uk for further information.

Infertility causes

There is no one definitive factor which causes infertility. According to the NHS, approximately one third of fertility problems are due to issues with the female, one third are down to problems with the male, and in up to 23% of circumstances doctors are unable to pinpoint a cause.

Infertility in women

Ovulation is vital to pregnancy, and without the monthly release of an egg there will be nothing for the male sperm to combine with. Failure to ovulate for whatever reason, is one of the most common causes of infertility and can occur as a result of a number of conditions:

Polycystic ovary syndrome (PCOS)

This is a condition that often inhibits the ovaries from producing an egg.

Early menopause (POI)

A women's ovaries stop working before she reaches the age of 40.

Thyroid problems

An underactive or overactive thyroid gland can prevent the occurrence of ovulation.

Chronic long-term illness

Some women who suffer from long-term chronic illnesses such as diabetes, cancer or kidney failure may not ovulate.

Cushing's syndrome

A hormonal disease that can stop the ovaries from releasing an egg.

Other possible causes of infertility in women include those listed below:

Problems with the womb or fallopian tubes

The fallopian tubes are essentially the pathway from the ovary to the womb, along which the egg travels whilst being fertilised along the way. When the egg reaches the end of its journey down the fallopian tubes, it is then implanted into the lining of the womb where it then grows and matures into a baby.

However, if either the fallopian tubes or the womb are damaged, or indeed if they stop working, it may then become very difficult to conceive.

Damage to the fallopian tubes or the womb can be caused by a number of factors. For example, pelvic surgery can sometimes scar the fallopian tubes, whilst cervical surgery can result in a shortening a the cervix (neck of the womb).

Pelvic inflammatory disease (PID)

This is an infection which occurs in areas including the fallopian tubes, womb and ovaries and is usually caused by a sexually transmitted infection (STI). The disease can damage and scar the fallopian tubes, thus meaning the egg is unable to travel into the womb.

Endometriosis

Endometriosis is a condition in which minute pieces of the womb lining begin to grow in other places, in the ovaries for example.

The growth of this sticky tissue or cysts can lead to blockages and misshaping of the pelvis and can also distort the way in which the follicle releases the egg.

Male infertility

For men, the most common cause of infertility is abnormal semen, accounting for 75% of all male infertility cases.

There are a number of explanations for abnormal male semen, some of which can be found listed below:

Low sperm count

Some men have a very low number of sperm, or in some cases they have none at all.

Low sperm mobility

This is where the sperm has difficulty making its way to the egg.

Abnormal sperm

In some cases, sperm may be an abnormal shape which makes it difficult for them to swim to the egg and fertilise it.

Other causes of male infertility include:

Testicles

The primary role of the testicles is to produce and store sperm, meaning that if they are damaged this can heavily impact the quality of semen. Damage can occur through infection, congenital defect, testicular cancer, injury, surgery, a lump in the testicles.

Ejaculation disorders

When a man ejaculates or 'comes' during sex, the sperm then travels up the cervix to gain access to the main part of the uterus and into the fallopian tubes. However, problems with ejaculation often means that the sperm is unable to do this.

⇨ Retrograde ejaculation is where the semen is ejaculated into the bladder, preventing it from taking the path it needs to in order to fertilise the egg.

⇨ Premature ejaculation is when ejaculation happens too fast. This is a relatively common condition which in many cases may not be so premature as to prevent conception. However, in cases where a man ejaculates before enough semen is deposited into the vagina, the migration of sperm to the fallopian tubes may be difficult.

Factors affecting both sexes

Age

Unfortunately age works against us if we are looking to conceive, and as we age our fertility begins to reduce.

According to statistics, the biggest drop in fertility levels occurs during our mid-thirties. For women who are aged 35, 95% will fall pregnant within three years of having regular unprotected sex. For women who are 38 however, this figure falls to 75%. Whilst fewer statistics exist with regards to male age and fertility, it is thought that men over the age of 35 are half as likely to achieve conception in comparison to men younger than 25.

Stress

Stress is a multi-faceted aspect of conception. There is a growing body of evidence suggesting that stress does in fact have a direct impact upon fertility – limiting the production of sperm in men, whilst also affecting ovulation within females.

In addition, many experts are also warning couples attempting to conceive about the indirect impact of stress. Work stress, for example, may have an effect upon partner relations, which can in turn lead to a reduction in libido which then leads to a reduced frequency of intercourse.

In addition, for couples who are desperately willing themselves to conceive, there is certainly a temptation to become an expert in the menstrual cycle, working out exactly when ovulation is occurring, keeping pregnancy tests stockpiled in the bathroom and having sex like it is a military operation. To either one partner, or both, making love may begin to simply feel like a routine, and subsequently resentment and stress may set in.

Weight

Being outside of a healthy weight range can seriously impact fertility. Women who are overweight or severely underweight for example, will often find that their ovulation is affected, or in some cases it may stop entirely.

Diagnosing infertility

Fertility testing and investigation can be a long and drawn out process from start to finish, so if you have reason to be concerned about conception then it is advisable for you to book an appointment with your GP as soon as possible.

Your GP will be able to give you advice about the next steps and will also carry out an assessment to explore possible areas of concern.

This will usually include your full medical, sexual and social history to help to identify what may be causing fertility problems. Your age, weight, length of time trying to conceive, and your sex life will usually be the starting points.

If it is a sexual problem this is usually easily dealt with. You will also typically be asked about medical conditions, sexually transmitted infections and menstrual cycle.

Some medications can affect your fertility, so your doctor may prescribe alternative treatments. Your GP will also ask you about smoking, being overweight or underweight, how much alcohol you drink and whether you take recreational drugs or have excessive stress in your life.

Infertility testing – the next steps

The doctor may also conduct a physical examination or refer you for further tests.

After your GP has considered your medical history and possibly carried out a physical examination, you may be referred to a specialist infertility team at an NHS hospital or fertility clinic for some further tests and procedures.

For women, there are a number of tests that can be used to try to establish the cause of infertility, including tests for Progesterone, Hormones, Thyroid and Chlamydia.

Other tests, including X-ray or ultrasound scan can detect any blockage of the fallopian tubes or problems around the cervix.

For men, a semen analysis and chlamydia test can be organised.

Should I tell my partner I am going to the doctor?

Yes, absolutely. If you have concerns about your fertility, talk to your partner – after all this is something which affects you both.

The thought that you may not be able to conceive may make it tempting to sneak off to visit your healthcare provider without another soul knowing, and whilst this is an understandable reaction it is always best to be open and honest about your concerns.

Tell your other half that you are worried and remember that fertility problems occur equally in men and women so both of you need to be there.

The realisation that there could in fact be an issue with conception can be an extremely emotional time, and certainly one in which both parties will need as much support from one another as possible.

⇨ The above information is reprinted with kind permission from the Counselling Directory. Please visit www.counselling-directory.org.uk for further information.

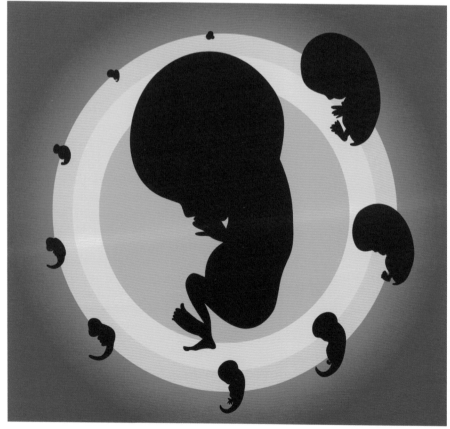

Young people 'missing out' on parenthood due to a lack of knowledge about their fertility

A survey of 1,000 young people from across the UK reveals worrying gaps in their knowledge of fertility and reproductive health, which experts believe may leave them ill-equipped to choose when to have children, prevent unplanned pregnancy or take steps to safeguard their fertility.

Around 80% of both sexes believe women's fertility only starts to decline after the age of 35, and a quarter of boys think women's fertility starts to decline after the age of 40, compared with 16% of girls. Two-thirds of those surveyed think men's fertility only starts declining after the age of 40, with a third believing it doesn't begin declining until after the age of 50. While the change is less dramatic for men, fertility rates for both sexes actually decline gradually from the late 20s, and can be affected by genetic and environmental factors such as smoking, obesity and nutrition.

Of the 16–24-year-olds surveyed, 94% of those who did not already have them said they would like to have children in the future. Of those who said they wanted children in the future, three-quarters of girls (76%) and two-thirds of boys (64%) said they would like to have children before they are 30. This is in stark contrast to the demographic shift upwards in the age of first birth in England and Wales – in 2014 for the first time over half (52%) of all births were to women aged 30 and over and two-thirds (67%) to men aged 30 and over. This is due to many factors including the socio-economic pressures of developing careers and establishing relationships.

These issues will be discussed at a Fertility Summit being held at the Royal College of Obstetricians and Gynaecologists today (Friday), convened by the British Fertility Society in partnership with the College and the Faculty of Sexual and Reproductive Healthcare.

The Summit aims to inspire debate and action on how to improve young people's knowledge of fertility and reproductive health, to ensure they are equipped with the right information to make informed decisions about their own fertility journey, or others they have an impact on. The event will hear from health and education professionals, as well as young people's groups and charities. Also speaking is the broadcaster Alex Jones, who is making a documentary about fertility and has spoken about the difficulties women face trying to balance their careers with motherhood.

Summit organiser Professor Adam Balen, Chair of the British Fertility Society, said: "The findings of this survey confirm our fears that many young people encounter few opportunities to learn about their reproductive health until they try to conceive. One in six couples experience difficulties in becoming pregnant and the associated emotional and physical impacts cannot be underestimated.

"Our aim is to ensure that the knowledge components of sex and relationship education not only cover how to avoid pregnancies and sexually transmitted infections, but also include information about fertility to help people plan. It should be choice not chance – we want to enable young people to make informed choices about pregnancy, whether that choice is to start a family or not."

Professor Lesley Regan, a fertility expert and Vice President for Strategic Development at the Royal College of Obstetricians and Gynaecologists, said: "While the risks should never be overplayed, men and women should be aware that reproductive outcomes are worse in older women. As well as it potentially taking longer to get pregnant, later maternity can involve a greater risk of miscarriage, a more complicated labour, and medical intervention at the birth.

"The wide range of social, professional and financial factors influencing the increasing age at which women are having their first baby is unlikely to be reversed dramatically, but it's important that both men and women are aware of when male and female fertility starts to decline.

"We also believe more should be done as a society to help people who would like to start a family earlier; for example, maternity pay, job security for women with young children, access to flexible working and the cost of childcare are all prohibitive factors to having children sooner."

Dr Chris Wilkinson, President of the Faculty of Sexual and Reproductive Healthcare and a consultant in sexual and reproductive healthcare, said: "The findings of this survey support the need for young people to be better informed about fertility and reproductive health. We remain concerned that sex and relationship education in schools is not universal. Where it does occur, this education can be variable and time spent on it is often very limited. We strongly urge governments across the UK to improve the quality of sex and relationship education so young people leave school armed with the necessary facts about not only safe sex, contraception and consent but also fertility and reproductive health."

Alex Jones, broadcaster and co-host of BBC's *The One Show*, said: "While exploring my own fertility and meeting couples experiencing fertility problems through making the documentary, I've been shocked by the amount of myths and misconceptions about fertility that contribute to a lack of awareness among both men and women. Infertility is heart breaking and I fully support anything that can be done to help educate young people about the facts to help them decide when, or if, to start a family."

Other findings from the survey:

⇨ The vast majority of young people – around nine in ten – are aware that women are most fertile under the age of 30

⇨ Encouragingly, 80% of girls and two-thirds of boys (66%) are aware that age is the number one factor which affects female fertility

⇨ Girls tend to consider that a higher number of factors affect their fertility than boys

⇨ Two-thirds of girls are now aware that being overweight or underweight affects fertility

⇨ 40% of girls mistakenly believe that having a miscarriage or being on the contraceptive pill for too long can adversely affect fertility

⇨ Substance abuse (drugs, alcohol, steroids) is perceived to be the main factor affecting male fertility – this does affect fertility but age remains the most common factor

⇨ Around 50% of young people did not recall seeing, hearing or talking about fertility in the past year

⇨ Of those that had, fewer than one in five recalled getting the info from official sources, such as through sex and relationship education, their GP or a sexual health clinic.

⇨ The above information is reprinted with kind permission from The Royal College of Gynaecologists. Please visit www.rcog.org.uk for further information.

Are you worried about your fertility? Young people share their stories

Rising house prices and financial instability are putting young people off starting families. But some fear they might be leaving it too late.

By Sarah Marsh

When do your chances of getting pregnant start to decline – late 20s, early 30s or after the age of 35? If your answer is the latter, you might be surprised to hear that in fact fertility rates for both men and women decline gradually from their late 20s.

Most people, however, are not aware of this. A poll, conducted to mark the Fertility Health summit, found worrying gaps in many 16- to 24-year-olds' knowledge of fertility and reproductive health.

The Guardian asked young readers about the subject, and we heard from lots of people who said that they couldn't even think about starting a family until they had a home and stable income – which tend to come much later for young adults today.

Aimee, 26, from Norwich said that money was a big factor: "We can't afford to buy a house and don't want to have a baby in rented accommodation because there's not enough security. Our landlord could decide to sell at any time."

But do young people still worry about their fertility? Here they share their stories.

Alex, 34: I wish I'd tried earlier – the ideal age for a man is your mid-20s

Like many men I assumed that there would not be any issue with my fertility. However, after two years of trying for a child, me and my partner got IVF. This revealed that I had low sperm motility, the most likely cause of our problems. We have since frozen some embryos so we can hopefully have another child in the future.

The clinic that we used made simple suggestions that improved my sperm motility significantly over a few months. I started drinking a lot more water and taking some vitamin supplements, which increased my sperm count and motility by 400%. By this point we had started the IVF process with success.

The ideal age to start trying is your mid-20s for a man, and early to mid-20s for a woman. However, it also depends on your relationship, emotional and financial stability, which now tend to come about towards the early to mid-30s. Therefore I think the only true answer can be that the ideal age differs for every individual based on these major factors.

Couples are now finding it much more difficult to find stable accommodation and incomes to be able to meet the demands of having a young family. The social welfare system is no longer the 'safety net' that it once was, in giving young couples the confidence that there is adequate social housing and benefits available for those struggling to get by.

Hattie, 29: Constant scaremongering does not help

I am not worried as such, however, as a 29-year-old single female, I have other people telling me that I should "start thinking about having a family" and get on with it.

As I am single at the moment and would like to be with someone for several years before starting said family then it is likely that I won't be trying until my early to mid-30s. I am hopeful that I will be able to get pregnant when I am ready, but have to face the possibility that my fertility or my partner's may be an issue, as we will be considered old parents.

However, I don't think constant scaremongering and pressure from the media and society in general helps.

Kylie, 25: My generation is really struggling

I worry about my fertility because I have polycystic ovary syndrome (PCOS) and am concerned that I will struggle to conceive. I have a long-term partner and we know we want children, but we are simply not in a financially stable enough position to do so yet. Hopefully we will be within the next few years, but I am worried it will keep being pushed back and we will run into problems.

Ideally I would have children around now as I feel both fit and healthy enough to have the best chance of a healthy pregnancy. I have the energy to run around after young children and I am at the peak of my fertility.

My generation are finding it takes longer to get established in a career, to save enough to buy a home, find a partner and settle down. There is also an attitude that careers need to come first – I particularly notice this among my male colleagues of a similar age, one of whom made a comment that a woman falling pregnant at this stage in her career would "have to get rid of it".

Nina, 34: I've made a lot of lifestyle changes to improve my chances

I have mild PCOS and started trying to get pregnant in January 2015, after being on the pill for 15 years. Nothing happened for six months and I went into a queue for an appointment with an NHS gynaecology consultant. After eight months of tests (blood, ultrasound and radiology), I was given the fertility drug Clomid. My husband was told he needed to change his lifestyle, so gave up smoking and cut back on beer.

Still nothing has happened but I have an increasing feeling of anxiety, pressure and a sense of doom. I'll be 35 in three months and my husband is 40, which doesn't help. The NHS does all it can with limited means. Private clinics charge high prices for alternative treatments such as acupuncture. Education is key:

reading up on lifestyle changes and alternative medicines helps to keep the anxiety at bay. Feeling impotent and powerless to kickstart the miracle of conception is all-consuming at times.

Aisha, 29: I used to worry about this, but then I learned to relax

My mother had lots of children, and didn't have the oldest until she was 30. I work in a scientific field and I used to be worried about fertility but recently was at a conference with lots of other female academics, all of whom were older than me. Both they and the people they work with all started their families at about 40 without a problem. This reassured me massively. Also, I'm not sure I even want children or if I'm feeling the pressure of expectation. If I didn't or couldn't have children my partner and I would be pragmatic enough to be OK with that.

I was panicking about being nearly 30 and not in any way ready for a baby (no house, no marriage, no permanent job). I was considering just having a baby right now, even though the timing would be entirely wrong. Now I'm a lot more relaxed. If I have a baby then great, if not then I'll find other things to do with my life instead.

I think the best age to have a child is between 32 and 35, depending on the individual. This is old enough to be in a stable career, to have a well-tested and stable relationship and to be in a decent house (owned or rented). You'll have had plenty of time for travelling, partying and everything else you might feel you've missed out on by having kids younger.

Kirsty, 34: Get fertility tests before it's too late

We have been trying for three years now to have a baby with no success and I have just been diagnosed with premature ovarian decline, meaning I've very few eggs left. It's heartbreaking.

We are both eating healthily and drinking less alcohol. I've changed my fitness regime and now have regular acupuncture. Life feels very much on hold at work and socially. I wish I'd frozen my eggs in my 20s.

The right time to have a baby is very individual but men and women should not take fertility for granted. It's important to be armed with information both in general terms and about your own individual profile. Get tests done before it's too late. Then you know if you can wait or if you should take some action, such as freezing eggs, if you haven't met the right person.

Education has prolonged the youth phase of life, and as social security and welfare become reduced and stigmatised people rightly want to be in a decent position to support a family before they have one. The housing situation also changes things – as average age at buying a first home rises, it's inevitable that having a family is put off too. These aren't choices so much as the effect of changing social and economic policies.

Neil, 34: My parents didn't have the luxury of living abroad

One of my brothers cannot have children and I worry that I have the same problem. That said, I am not at the stage where I want to have children, although I realise time is running out. I think that the ideal age to have a child is probably 32, that means you have had time to enjoy your 20s and to mature.

Young people are choosing to have children later because our options are very different. My parents would never have had the luxury of having the choice to live abroad, take time to travel or even study at university. Rural Ireland in my parents' generation was a different world (and one where contraception was illegal).

20 April 2016

⇨ The above information is reprinted with kind permission from *The Guardian*. Please visit www.theguardian.com for further information.

Over half of younger women with breast cancer "in the dark" about preserving fertility

Despite NICE guidance recommending fertility options be offered to young women facing cancer treatment, just over half (53%) of younger women diagnosed with breast cancer have no discussion with healthcare professionals about fertility preservation options, including freezing embryos or eggs, according to new findings from Breast Cancer Care.

Shockingly, this is despite National Institute for Health and Care Excellence (NICE) guidelines recommending women of reproductive age are offered fertility preservation before starting breast cancer treatment.

The majority (86%) of almost 500 younger women surveyed by Breast Cancer Care said they received chemotherapy, a treatment that can cause infertility. The survey also revealed more than a quarter (28%) of younger women with breast cancer would like to have a child or add to their family after treatment.

The charity is concerned that younger women with breast cancer are being denied the chance to make an informed decision about trying to preserve their fertility. This includes egg or embryo freezing.

Naomi Sneade, 32, from Bournemouth, was diagnosed with breast cancer in 2012 when she was 29, and then her cancer came back at the end of 2014. She says:

"There was so much information to take in after my breast cancer diagnosis. I was told the chemotherapy I needed could affect my fertility, that there was a drug that could protect my ovaries and then it was on to the next step.

"There was no discussion about fertility preservation and I didn't even realise there were options until I met other young women who talked about freezing their eggs and embryos. I've always seen having kids in my future and now I worry I've missed the chance to try and preserve my fertility. This is devastating.

"So when my cancer came back a year ago, fertility was my first question, instead of my last. But sadly no one can answer whether I'll be able to start a family."

Samia al Qadhi, Chief Executive of Breast Cancer Care, says:

"These worrying findings suggest younger women with breast cancer are being left in the dark. They are not getting the chance to talk about preserving their fertility alongside treating the cancer.

"On top of being told you have breast cancer, chemotherapy can shatter young women's hopes of a family. After diagnosis there is a short window of opportunity to try and preserve fertility.

"So we are calling for shared responsibility between healthcare professionals to ensure younger women with breast cancer have the conversation they deserve about fertility preservation options as early as possible. While fertility preservation may not be wanted by everyone, it is extremely important for thousands of younger women with breast cancer."

Breast Cancer Care is calling for improved communication between breast and fertility clinics. The charity has also developed a new Fertility Toolkit for setting up a fertility referral pathway for young women with breast cancer at the point of diagnosis. This will help ensure they are given the choice to have a discussion with a fertility specialist.

Anyone looking for support can visit breastcancercare.org.uk or call the Helpline on 0808 800 6000 from day one.

⇨ The above information is reprinted with kind permission from Breast Cancer Care. Please visit www.breastcancercare.org.uk for further information.

© Breast Cancer Care 2017

Smartphone app could allow men to test their fertility at home

Gadget designed to clip onto a smartphone able to detect abnormal sperm samples with 98% accuracy in trials.

Men may soon be able to measure their own sperm count and quality at home, using a smartphone app developed by scientists.

In early tests, the gadget, designed to clip onto a smartphone, detected abnormal sperm samples with an accuracy of 98%.

In more than 40% of cases where couples struggle to conceive, the underlying fertility issue is linked to sperm abnormalities, but the researchers said that social stigma and lack of access to testing meant than many men never seek evaluation.

Hadi Shafiee, who led the work at Brigham and Women's Hospital in Boston, US, said: "We wanted to come up with a solution to make male infertility testing as simple and affordable as home pregnancy tests."

The team put the device together using spare parts from DVD and CD drives at a total cost of $4.45. Using the device simply involves drawing semen into a disposable holder that is plugged into one side of the phone attachment, in a similar way to a USB.

In seconds, results of the analysis are displayed on the phone's screen.

In the study, published in the journal *Science Translational Medicine*, the research team recruited 10 volunteers with no formal training, including administrative assistants employed at a Boston fertility clinic. They correctly classified more than 100 semen samples using the app.

Overall, the scientists examined 350 clinic samples and were able to identify those with low sperm counts and inactive or poorly motile sperm with 98% accuracy.

John Petrozza, director of the Massachusetts General Hospital Fertility Center and a co-author, described the device as a "true game-changer". "Men have to provide semen samples in these rooms at a hospital, a situation in which they often experience stress, embarrassment, pessimism and disappointment," he said.

"Current clinical tests are lab-based, time-consuming and subjective. This test is low-cost, quantitative, highly accurate and can analyse a video of an undiluted, unwashed semen sample in less than five seconds."

Allan Pacey, professor of andrology at the University of Sheffield, who was not involved in the research, said that the techniques used for sperm quality assessment have not changed significantly since the 1950s, and that even when carried out at specialist centres can be prone to errors if the laboratory worker has not had sufficient training.

"As such, the development of an easy, cheap and accurate method to evaluate the sperm present in a sample of semen would be very welcome, particularly if it could be carried out by someone without specific training and in any location," he said.

However, he added that the smartphone device could not replicate all the tests carried out in a specialist lab and did not analyse morphology – sperm size and shape.

"For a small number of men whose sperm are badly made, and have poor morphology, it would be important to get this diagnosed correctly," he said. "So any man who struggles with infertility for a significant length of time, say more than 12 months, should consider getting their test repeated in a specialist laboratory, regardless of what the phone app might have concluded."

The team behind the device are planning to perform additional testing and will file for approval from the FDA, the US regulator.

22 March 2017

⇨ The above information is reprinted with kind permission from *The Guardian*. Please visit www.theguardian.com for further information.

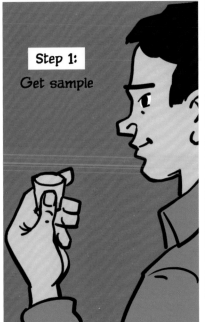

Step 1:
Get sample

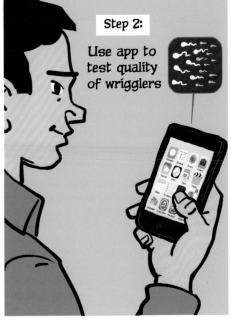

Step 2:
Use app to test quality of wrigglers

"Why aren't you pregnant yet?" – the questions infertile women dread

Many young women receive intrusive questions and remarks about when they might get pregnant. Laura Cooke describes how that feels for women who can't have the families they would like.

By Laura Cooke

I'm sitting in a car with a male colleague, heading back from a meeting. I don't know him that well but we're having a pleasant conversation about life and love, filling in the blanks about the other's background. Talk turns to my recent wedding. And then he hits me with this question: "Are you going to have kids?"

I consider giving him a noncommittal "not yet" or "maybe". But instead I decide to tell him the truth – that I am infertile. I had both my fallopian tubes and ovaries removed at the age of 30. As my ovaries were turning gangrenous, I had little choice in the matter.

He is slightly taken aback by my answer but we discuss it further. He says he admires my honesty and the conversation moves on.

At the time, and in the context of the conversation, it didn't strike me as an odd question. But in retrospect, it's a hugely personal question, and potentially quite an offensive one, to ask someone whose history is unknown to you.

According to the NHS, one in seven couples may have difficulty conceiving. This is approximately 3.5 million people in the UK.

So bearing that figure in mind, why do people persist in asking women in long-term relationships about their plans to start a family? "Are you pregnant? Why not? When are you going to have children? Aren't you leaving it a bit late? Time is running out!"

I can appreciate it would be an irritating line of questioning for a woman who is childless through choice. For someone like me who has had it forced upon them, it is downright heartbreaking. Considering as a nation

we still struggle to talk about difficult subjects, it's odd that we are so willing to ask near strangers such intimate questions and even more bizarre that those being asked feel obliged to answer and explain ourselves.

I think part of the reason it is seen as acceptable is that society sees other people's lives, and women's bodies, as public property. We share everything on Facebook – wedding photos, food porn, holiday plans and, yes, baby scans. Certain publications are awash with regular 'is she or isn't she' pregnancy speculation (a recent example being the _Daily Mail_'s hard-hitting article on whether Jennifer Aniston was harbouring a big lunch or a new life). And of course this inevitably spills over into 'real life'.

Although we have thankfully come a long way since women were shunned for having a child out of wedlock, the traditional view that starting a family is the next logical step after a woman gets married, particularly to a man, is still alive and well in 2016, as demonstrated by my well-meaning colleague. With women often reluctant to talk about fertility problems, through shame, embarrassment, pride or whatever reason, the people who ask them these intrusive questions aren't called out on it.

As crap as my fertility situation is, in a funny kind of way I feel fortunate that at least I know I am infertile. Without medical help, nothing short of a Biblical miracle will see life spring from my loins. I know why my reproductive system won't work – because half of it is AWOL.

And I also feel fortunate that I am able to talk to people about it, tell them my story, thus heading off many of the questions people think it is acceptable to ask women of childbearing age.

Perhaps this is my way of taking back control of the situation, following my abrupt crash into infertility.

But it's far from being that cut and dried for many couples experiencing fertility issues. I know couples who are, on the face of it, healthy people, but after years of trying to conceive naturally and years of treatment, they still haven't succeeded. After years of highly invasive tests, the consultant still hasn't got a clue why this couple cannot make a baby.

Toni Gardner spent eight years trying to conceive with husband Derek before finally falling pregnant through IVF treatment.

Toni, who runs the Treelight Fertility Support Group in East Sussex, spent those eight years fending off insensitive comments from friends, family and co-workers, who had no idea of her inner turmoil.

She said, "I used to hear 'tick tock tick tock', 'come on, you two have been together long enough now'. And 'your ovaries aren't going to stay young forever, don't you think it's about time you started having children?' Then I had family members saying 'I had children by the time I was 23, you're 31 now,' blah blah blah.

"The one thing that really hurt me was I overheard people talking at a party. Two people were talking and one said 'Have Toni and Derek got any kids?' and the other person said 'No not yet I think Toni is focused on her career.'"

Toni, a qualified therapist, didn't feel able to talk about the difficulties she was facing, hoping instead that people would just get the hint. She said, "A lot of the time when people said to me 'When are you going to have kids?' I used to say 'Believe me, I'm trying,' and people used to say 'Come on Toni, it's been forever.' So I would fix them with a steely gaze and repeat 'Believe me, I'm trying,' and keep looking at them and hope they would get the hint. Sometimes they did, sometimes they didn't."

So should we just carry on like this, dropping vague hints in the hope that the person asking the question will understand the topic is out of bounds? Or should we be more proactive and start a conversation about infertility and attempt to educate people that badgering women about babies is not OK?

On the back of her experiences, Toni Gardner set up a support group for women experiencing fertility issues because she says she couldn't bear the thought of anyone suffering by themselves.

She is also currently writing a book based on some of the insensitive comments she had to endure during those eight years.

This article is my own small way of putting the message out there: stop asking women about their pregnancy plans. That woman in the office who cried this morning when her period started? She doesn't need your insensitive comments. Your friend? She has just had her third early miscarriage. She doesn't want to hear your opinion on her ovaries.

And as for the next person who hits me with that 'tick tock' nonsense…have I ever shown you my oophorectomy scars…?

19 August 2016

⇨ The above information is reprinted with kind permission from The F Word. Please visit www.thefword. org.uk for further information.

Stages of grief in infertility

By Francine Blanchet

The issues that face those with infertility problems may include any number of emotional responses including fear that they are "not normal", loss of self-esteem and/or a sense that they are not in control of the direction of their lives. They may also face existential anxieties regarding the purpose of their lives – "What am I here for?" or, "How do I now define myself in the world?". A fear that stretches ahead of them with no children to occupy their time and energy. They may ask themselves, "What do I do with my life if they are no children?"

Denial

People who receive a diagnostic of infertility typically respond with shock and denial. It can take time before one can accept the reality of their situation. The refusal is normally a state that does not last long, it is a state of shock. One cannot work their head around the situation and accept the medical position that there is something wrong, especially if the couple had dreams about having a child and a family.

Anger

The couple now need to deal with the loss – the loss of the dream, the loss of an imagined future, the loss of being unable to procreate, the loss of being a biological parent. The anger can be distributed widely including being irrational with staff and colleagues at work and even exhibiting irritation with everybody at the infertility clinic. They can say that those who are trying to help are incompetent, didn't do enough, that they have not proven themselves. The client is not conscious of that. They believe they are in their right to complain and to react the way they do. It is also difficult when they are through this stage and the couple are trying to understand each other's grief. Nobody mourns in the same way so instead of helping each other, they can be pushing each other away.

Fences are erected and there is a desire sometimes to hurt each other because of the hurt the client is experiencing. It is a complex emotion and sometimes we just need to react to this in a sensitive way.

Bargaining

This is when the client wants to exert control over the situation. In their mind there is a process of give and take. "If I could get pregnant just once, I promise I would be the best parent ever. I only ask for one child and I will start to give my time to some charities".

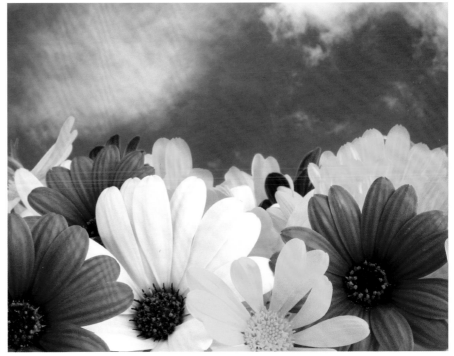

Or just getting pregnant to know how it feels. It is a very painful process when it does not work, because the bargaining never works. The couple can revert to anger very easily.

Depression

Over time many couples find that they begin to despair of achieving their goal of having their own biological child. An infertile person may become depressed. It might be overwhelming as they face the possibility that the child they were striving to have may never be.

When the couple confronts their fears of being childless, the anxiety and the tension can increase.

It is important to distinguish between sadness as a healthy response to a major shift in one's self-image and sense of one's place in the world, which requires recognition, time and understanding to work through, as opposed to depression which is a more sustained response. Depression needs long-term management to resolve. (Stuck grief will be discussed later).

The loss attached to childlessness may include loss of faith, loss of power, loss of dreams in the future and loss of sexuality and intimacy. Then for the male, it is the loss of self-image (virility) and for the women, not being a true 'women' and being able to fulfil that function properly. The couple feels they have failed the basic task, having a family.

Acceptance

This can be defined at the point which the person has accepted the reality of the loss and then are able to put energy into the present and to start to plan for the future. It can emerge at any stage of the infertility treatment or management process. Couples may come to accept that they will never have a child and feel able, even eager to move forward to a new life without children. They come to an acceptance of their infertility and feel ready to consider the option of donated sperms or ovaries to help them to have a child within their relationship. The infertile couple needs to accept that they will not have the imagined child of the relationship and be ready to incorporate a different way of creating a family.

At this time the person or the couple will have grieved the loss of their fertility, as well as the loss of their biological child. They will be prepared to move on with renewed energy to the acceptance of a child through adoption or gamete donation. Acceptance may be indicated to take up a treatment option that previously had been unacceptable to them.

What is there to do?

Worden's four tasks of mourning:

⇨ Acknowledge the reality of the situation – it is important after having experienced denial that the loss is fully acknowledged. The client may discount the significance of the loss, the infertile person may search for another diagnostic or may be unable to let go of a scan picture of the implanted embryo.

⇨ Work through the pain of grief – some people will not allow themselves to feel at all and focus on the next treatment. One of the aims of grief counselling is to help facilitate people through this difficult task so they don't carry the pain throughout their life. Sooner or later, some of those who avoid all conscious grieving, break down – usually with some form of depression. The unseen nature of infertility means that it is all the more easy for those around them to discount their pain and to try to point out all the positive sides of child-free living, at the time where the couple needs to feel that they are allowed to cry, rage and feel the pain of this enormous blow to their sense of themselves, their hope and their aspirations.

⇨ Adjust to the environment – this is the last part of the acceptation.

⇨ Emotionally relocate and move on with life – reinvent their life without children and take pleasure and meaning in the world where their own biological children are missing.

Egan helping model:

Firstly, exploration: taking time to look at what is there – resources, passion and hobbies to be built upon those so to help for a new meaning. The second stage is new understanding: there is hope and after the bereavement and the sadness, some actions can be taken. Finally, action: start with taking care of the body, possibly exercising, eating well and meeting friends.

10 February 2016

⇨ The above information is reprinted with kind permission from Counselling Directory. Please visit www.counselling-directory.org.uk for further information.

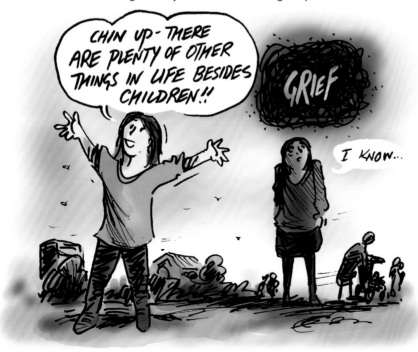

Feelings after pregnancy loss

Reading how other people have felt may help you feel less alone. You will almost certainly find that some people have had similar feelings to yours, and that can be reassuring.

But the experience of miscarriage is different for everyone. What the loss of your baby means to you, and how you feel about it, will be shaped by all kinds of things to do with the person you are and your particular circumstances. So, although you will probably find you share a lot with others, it's important to remember that no one else's experience of miscarriage will be exactly like yours.

Here is what some people have said:

"I've never cried so much in my whole life. I was walking about with an empty feeling where I should have been holding my baby."

"I keep on thinking it's a punishment. I must have done something wrong."

"I've got such a mad mixture of emotions – grief, guilt, anger, fear but also relief that my wife isn't in pain any more."

"I went to the hospital and had a check over and was sent home with nothing more than an empty feeling. I wasn't told that I would keep bleeding or feel so crappy, I wasn't told how difficult it would be to deal with and process."

"After the operation [for an ectopic pregnancy] I was in complete shock. I had just found out I was pregnant and then it was suddenly all over. Not only had I lost the baby but I also felt physically damaged. Afterwards I focused on recovering physically, but emotionally I was completely numb."

"I wasn't sure if I was pregnant, so when it happened it was a shock and a relief at the time. After a few days I just carried on as normal."

"My mother was relieved, I also didn't tell her until a few weeks after the miscarriage and she was positive, said it was for the best. I know why she felt that way but it still hurt. Those around me made me feel like I had no right to be upset about this. I'm pretty sure they didn't mean to, but I was absolutely devastated and I don't think anyone understood why."

Your feelings

A miscarriage is not a major event for everyone, but it is for many women –

and men too. Most people are left with feelings of great sadness and regret. You might feel shocked and confused. You may feel angry – at fate, at your partner, at other women who seem to have no problems getting and staying pregnant.

You might feel guilty and wonder whether you have been responsible for your loss in some way (that's very unlikely). You may just feel empty and perhaps lonely. Some women lose confidence, feel stressed, panicky and out of control.

If you didn't plan the pregnancy or if you didn't want to be pregnant, you may find it hard to understand your emotions. You might feel completely different to the way you thought you would. You might feel a mixture of loss, relief and guilt.

Many women – and partners too – find it difficult to be around anyone else who is pregnant or has a new baby. It's certainly very common to feel jealous and to feel that this is all very unfair.

For some people, their feelings are intense but not overwhelming. Others are devastated by what they feel and for a time feel barely able to cope. Everyday tasks, whether at home or at work, can seem impossible to manage or not worth doing. The world can feel turned upside down.

You may find it helpful to read our leaflet *Your feelings after miscarriage*. You might also find it helpful to use our online forum, where you can share your thoughts and feelings with others.

Our personal reflections section is another place where you can find a range of writing from people who have been through pregnancy loss. Natasza's story, for example, captures her feelings of grief, loss and isolation after her loss.

Physical feelings

It is also common to feel loss in physical ways. A lot of women find they feel very tired, even some time after the miscarriage. You may also have headaches or stomach-aches, be constipated, have diarrhoea, or find it hard to sleep. These symptoms will probably disappear in time, but if you feel worried about them, it might be a good idea to talk to your GP.

Your partner's feelings

Partners too can have strong feelings of loss, distress and anxiety, yet their needs

can go unrecognised. They may find it helpful to read our leaflet *Partners Too* (or an earlier version *Men and Miscarriage*) and/or the web-based article "Coping with miscarriage".

If you haven't been able to tell your family, friends or partner about your miscarriage – or if you don't have a partner – then you may feel very lonely and isolated. You might find it helpful to look at our information on talking about miscarriage.

A particular kind of loss

Miscarriage is a particular kind of loss and can bring particular feelings.

After a miscarriage, you grieve for a person you never knew, and for a relationship that ended before it really began. You grieve not for a person who has lived and died but for the hopes and plans and dreams that you had for your baby and your family. You grieve for the loss of your future as the parent of this baby. You are sad not just because of what you have lost but because of what will never be.

This is different to grieving for, say, an elderly person who has died, and it can be hard for people who have no experience of miscarriage to understand.

Another way in which grief after the loss of a baby is different to other kinds of grief is that you might be thinking about the possibility of another pregnancy in the future. So your feelings about what has happened may be mixed with anxieties about why it happened, whether and when you might conceive again, and if you do conceive, whether you might lose the next baby too.

Sometimes the words 'loss' and 'losing' don't feel right. You might think that 'losing a baby' sounds like something to be blamed for, as if you were careless. That's certainly not what we mean when we use these words.

⇨ The above information is reprinted with kind permission from the Miscarriage Association. Please visit www.miscarriageassociation.org.uk for further information.

Treatments for infertility

There are many different treatments for infertility available that can increase your chances of getting pregnant (conceiving). So it's worth seeking help if you're having trouble conceiving. Some couples take two years or more to get pregnant naturally. But if you and your partner haven't conceived after a year of regular sex and no contraception, it could be a sign of fertility problems.

How can I boost my fertility?

There are some things you can do to help you to conceive naturally. If you see your GP because you're having trouble getting pregnant, they'll usually talk you through these first.

Sticking to a healthy lifestyle may improve your chances of getting pregnant and having a healthy baby. So, quit smoking or at least cut down, and check your alcohol intake too. Both men and women shouldn't drink more than 14 units a week on a regular basis. And if you're trying for a baby (as well as if you get pregnant), guidelines from the UK Chief Medical Officers are that it's best for women not to drink alcohol at all. Maintaining a healthy weight may also help, because being either overweight or underweight can affect your fertility.

Eating a balanced and varied diet should help you get all the nutrients your body needs. But women who are planning a pregnancy should take folic acid and vitamin D supplements. Speak to your pharmacist about which supplements you can take safely before and during pregnancy. See our Related information for more about healthy eating when planning a pregnancy.

Having sex every two to three days will help to make sure you're having sex around the time of ovulation (a woman's most fertile time of the month). This will maximise your chances of conceiving. If you use lubricants, be aware that some of these can affect the quality of a man's sperm and make them less likely to fertilise an egg.

When to seek help for fertility problems

Seeing a GP

More than eight out of ten couples will conceive within one year of having regular, unprotected sex. If you've been trying for a year, it might be worth seeing your GP for advice. Think about seeing your GP sooner than this if you're a woman aged over 35. Your GP will be able to talk through things you can try to boost your fertility. They may also be able to do some initial investigations, such as testing for ovulation in women and a semen analysis in men.

Referral to a specialist

For further tests and treatments for infertility, you'll need to be referred to a specialist0 fertility doctor. The criteria for when you can be referred to specialist fertility services on the NHS may vary between different regions. It's usually only after you've been trying to conceive for at least a year with regular sex and no contraception, but this depends on your age, your tests results and local guidelines.

You may be referred sooner if you're a woman over the age of 35, f initial test results have shown up something abnormal, or if your infertility is thought to be linked to a specific cause. Once you've got a referral, you may have to wait for treatment, and NHS waiting lists vary from area to area. Even if you're eligible for treatment on the NHS, you'll still need to pay the normal prescription charges for any fertility medicines you're prescribed.

Getting private treatment

You can choose to have infertility treatments privately, which means you have to pay the costs yourself. The costs vary from one clinic to another. Before accepting any treatments privately, you should be given a personalised treatment plan outlining all of the costs involved.

At a specialist fertility clinic, you'll be offered an assessment, followed by tests and treatments if these are appropriate for you. It's important to choose a clinic that's right for you, so take your time over your decision. Check which services clinics offer, your eligibility for their treatment, and their location, opening hours and waiting times. Some clinics have age and weight (or body mass index) restrictions on patients. Some will only treat you privately. The success rates between clinics vary too.

Fertility drugs

Women

Your doctor may be able to prescribe some medicines to improve your fertility and increase your chances of getting pregnant.

Women who aren't ovulating regularly or at all, may be able to take medicines that stimulate their ovaries to make eggs. This is called ovulation induction. Clomifene citrate is often the first medicine that doctors recommend. You can use clomifene for up to six months, but if the medicine is going to work, this usually happens within around three months. Clomifene can cause hot flushes, mood swings, depression and headaches. It's important to discuss all of the possible side-effects with your doctor before you start any treatment.

If clomifene hasn't worked for you, your doctor may recommend gonadotrophin injections instead. These also trigger ovulation. There are also other medicines (for example, tamoxifen) which stimulate your ovaries. If you have polycystic ovary syndrome, which can affect ovulation, your doctor may prescribe a medicine called metformin. You may take metformin with clomifene or on its own.

Medicines that stimulate your ovaries (such as the ones mentioned above) are associated with a higher risk of multiple pregnancy.

Men

Low testosterone levels in men (called hypogonadism) can affect sperm production and sperm quality. If you have this condition, your doctor may suggest you try gonadotrophin injections. These work by triggering your body to make testosterone.

If you have retrograde ejaculation, your sperm are ejaculated backwards into your bladder instead of through your urethra to the outside of your body. Medicines that close the opening to your bladder, such as pseudoephedrine, may help.

Medicines such as sildenafil (Viagra) may be helpful if you have trouble getting an erection.

Surgery for infertility

Depending on what's causing your infertility, your doctor may recommend surgery. If so, you will be referred to a surgeon to discuss your options.

Women

For women who have polycystic ovary syndrome and have already tried clomifene, a type of surgery called laparoscopic ovarian drilling may help. This keyhole surgery technique can stimulate your ovaries to ovulate (release eggs). During surgery, your surgeon will make tiny holes in the surface of your ovary.

Women who have a small blockage in one of their fallopian tubes may be able to have surgery to clear it. Sometimes, scar tissue in your uterus can stop you having periods and getting pregnant. If this is the case, the tissue needs to be removed.

If you have endometriosis, tissue from the lining of your uterus grows in other places in your body. This may affect your fertility. Your doctor may recommend you have surgery to remove or destroy this extra tissue.

Men

Surgery can also help some men with fertility problems. You may have a blockage in the tubes that take sperm from your testicles to your penis or in your epididymis, which stores sperm. If this is what's causing your problems, you may be able to have an operation to remove the blockage and restore your fertility.

If you have varicoceles (swollen veins in your scrotum) and no other reason for your infertility has been found, your doctor may suggest surgery. Surgery for varicoceles is thought to improve quality of your sperm, but there's no evidence that it will increase your chance of having a baby. If this treatment is an option, your doctor will discuss this further with you.

Assisted conception

If other treatments don't work, or aren't appropriate for you, your doctor may recommend that you try assisted conception (assisted reproduction). These procedures control the way your sperm and egg are brought together so that you're more likely to conceive.

The three main types of assisted conception are intra-uterine insemination (IUI), in vitro fertilisation (IVF) and intracytoplasmic sperm injection (ICSI). You may be able to use your own sperm or eggs or donor sperm or eggs, depending on what's causing your infertility.

Intra-uterine insemination (IUI)

IUI involves taking a sample of sperm and placing it inside the woman's uterus close to the time of ovulation. It's useful for men who have ejaculation problems or mild problems with the quality of their sperm.

IUI is usually combined with injections to stimulate the woman's ovaries. This may cause several eggs to develop at the same time, which can lead to a multiple pregnancy (twins, triplets or more).

In vitro fertilisation (IVF)

IVF involves removing one or more of the woman's eggs and mixing them with sperm in a laboratory. Once the eggs are fertilised (usually after two or three days), the embryos (fertilised eggs) are placed in the woman's uterus. The woman may need to take medicines to stimulate her ovaries to produce several eggs at once. This is called superovulation and increases your chances of a pregnancy.

A doctor may suggest IVF for women who have blocked fallopian tubes or if other treatments, such as fertility drugs, haven't worked. It may also be suggested if you have endometriosis. IVF may also be recommended if men have ejaculation problems or mild problems with the quality of their sperm. It's also the recommended procedure if a cause can't be found for your infertility (called unexplained infertility).

Intracytoplasmic sperm injection (ICSI)

In ICSI, a single sperm is injected directly into an egg in a laboratory. This means that only a very small number of sperm are needed to be sure of fertilising the egg. The resulting embryo is transferred to the woman's uterus.

ICSI is used if a man has a very low sperm count or abnormal sperm. Sperm may be collected directly from his testicles or epididymis.

Complications of assisted conception

Having fertility treatment makes you more likely to have a multiple pregnancy (such as twins or triplets). This is why there are strict restrictions on how many embryos can be transferred into your uterus at one time. A multiple pregnancy increases the risk of health problems for you and your babies. You may be more likely to have a miscarriage, premature birth and high blood pressure.

Your body can over-react to the medicines used to stimulate your ovaries. This can cause ovarian hyperstimulation syndrome (OHSS). Around one in four women develop mild OHSS. If you have mild OHSS, you may have a bloated tummy and feel sick. In fewer than eight in every 100 IVF cycles, women develop severe OHSS, which can cause serious health problems. Contact your fertility clinic straightaway if you:

⇨ feel sick or vomit

⇨ have severe pain in your tummy

⇨ notice any swelling in your tummy

⇨ feel short of breath or faint

⇨ suddenly put on a lot of weight.

Your risk of having an ectopic pregnancy (when your baby grows outside your uterus) may be higher if you have IVF or other assisted conception treatments.

Removing the eggs for IVF or ICSI involves passing a needle through your vagina and into your ovary. This can cause an infection. If this happens, you'll usually be given antibiotics.

Babies conceived by IVF may have a low birth weight or be born early in pregnancy. There has been some research to suggest that fertility treatment may be associated with a higher risk of birth defects. However, the risk of this happening is very low – the majority of babies conceived this way are not affected. It may be that any increased risk is related to the infertility problems in the parents, rather than the treatment itself.

Last updated May 2017

⇨ The above information is reprinted with kind permission from Bupa. Please visit www.bupa.co.uk for further information.

IVF – what is in vitro fertilisation (IVF) and how does it work?

What is IVF?

In vitro fertilisation (IVF) literally means 'fertilisation in glass'.

IVF treatment involves the fertilisation of an egg (or eggs) outside the body. The treatment can be performed using your own eggs and sperm, or using either donated sperm or donated eggs, or both.

A clinic may recommend IVF if:

⇨ you have been diagnosed with unexplained infertility

⇨ your fallopian tubes are blocked

⇨ other techniques such as fertility drugs or intrauterine insemination (IUI) have not been successful

⇨ the male partner has fertility problems but not severe enough to require intra-cytoplasmic sperm injection (ICSI)

⇨ you are using your partner's frozen sperm in your treatment and IUI is not suitable for you

⇨ you are using donated eggs or your own frozen eggs in your treatment

⇨ you are using embryo testing to avoid passing on a genetic condition to your child.

How does IVF work?

IVF techniques vary according to your individual circumstances and the approach of your clinic. Before your treatment starts, you will need to complete various consent forms. You and, if applicable, your partner may also need to have blood tests to screen for HIV, hepatitis B, hepatitis C and human T cell lymphotropic virus (HTLV) I and II.

Treatment then typically involves the following stages:

For women:

1. Suppressing your natural monthly hormone cycle

As a first step you will be given a drug to suppress your natural cycle, which you can administer yourself in the form of a daily injection or a nasal spray. The drug treatment continues for about two weeks.

2. Boosting the egg supply

After your natural cycle has been suppressed, you will be given a type of fertility hormone known as a gonadotrophin. You will usually take this as a daily injection for around 12 days. The hormone will increase the number of eggs you produce.

3. Checking on progress

The clinic will monitor your progress throughout the drug treatment through vaginal ultrasound scans and, possibly, blood tests. Between 34 and 38 hours before your eggs are due to be collected you will be given a hormone injection to help your eggs mature. This is likely to be human chorionic gonadotrophin (hCG).

4. Collecting the eggs

Your eggs will usually be collected using ultrasound guidance while you are sedated. A hollow needle is attached to the ultrasound probe and is used to collect the eggs from the follicles on each ovary. You may experience some cramps, feel a little sore and bruised and/or experience a small amount of bleeding from the vagina. After your eggs have been collected, you will be given medication in the form of pessaries, injection or gel to help prepare the lining of your womb for embryo transfer.

5. Fertilising the eggs

Your eggs will be mixed with your partner's or the donor's sperm and cultured in the laboratory for 16–20 hours after which they are checked for signs of fertilisation.

Those that have been fertilised (now called embryos) will be grown in the laboratory incubator for up to six days. The embryologist will monitor the development of the embryos and the best will then be chosen for transfer. Any remaining embryos of suitable quality can be frozen for future use.

6. Embryo transfer

If you are under the age of 40, one or two embryos may be transferred. If you are 40 or over, a maximum of three may be used.

The number of embryos transferred is restricted because of the risks associated with multiple births. Due to this, your clinic will recommend single embryo transfer (SET) if they feel it is the best option for you.

During the procedure, a doctor or nurse will insert a speculum into your vagina. This is similar to having a cervical smear taken, when a speculum is used to hold the vagina open so the cervix is visible.

A fine tube (catheter) is then passed through the cervix, normally using ultrasound guidance. The embryos are passed down the tube into the womb.

This is normally a pain-free procedure and usually no sedation is necessary, but you may experience a little discomfort because you need a full bladder if ultrasound is used.

For men:

Around the time your partner's eggs are collected, you will be asked to produce a sample of sperm.

The sperm will be washed and prepared so the active, normal sperm are separated from the poorer-quality sperm.

If you have stored sperm, it will be removed from frozen storage, thawed and prepared in the same way.

⇨ The above information is reprinted with kind permission from the Human Fertilisation & Embryology Authority. Please visit www.hfea.gov.uk for further information.

© Human Fertilisation & Embryology Authority 2017

IVF – availability

Who can have IVF?

IVF is only offered on the NHS if certain criteria are met. If you don't meet these criteria, you may need to pay for private treatment.

NICE recommendations

In 2013, the National Institute for Health and Care Excellence (NICE) published new fertility guidelines that made recommendations about who should have access to IVF treatment on the NHS in England and Wales.

However, individual NHS Clinical Commissioning Groups (CCGs) make the final decision about who can have NHS-funded IVF in their local area, and their criteria may be stricter than those recommended by NICE (see below).

Women under 40

According to NICE, women aged under 40 should be offered three cycles of IVF treatment on the NHS if:

⇨ they've been trying to get pregnant through regular unprotected sex for two years, or

⇨ they've not been able to get pregnant after 12 cycles of artificial insemination.

If you turn 40 during treatment, the current cycle will be completed, but further cycles should not be offered.

If tests show that IVF is the only treatment likely to help you get pregnant, you should be referred for IVF straight away.

Women aged 40 to 42

The NICE guidelines also say that women aged 40 to 42 should be offered one cycle of IVF on the NHS if all of the following four criteria are met:

⇨ they've been trying to get pregnant through regular unprotected sex for two years, or haven't been able to get pregnant after 12 cycles of artificial insemination

⇨ they've never had IVF treatment before

⇨ they show no evidence of low ovarian reserve (where eggs in your ovaries are low in number or quality)

⇨ they have been informed of the additional implications of IVF and pregnancy at this age.

Again, if tests show that IVF is the only treatment likely to help you get pregnant, you should be referred for IVF straight away.

IVF on the NHS

NHS trusts across England and Wales are working to provide the same levels of service. However, the provision of IVF treatment varies across the country and often depends on local CCG policies.

CCGs may have additional criteria you need to meet before you can have IVF on the NHS, such as:

⇨ not having any children already, from both your current and any previous relationships

⇨ being a healthy weight

⇨ not smoking

⇨ falling into a certain age range (for example, some CCGs only fund treatment for women under 35).

In some cases, only one cycle of IVF may be routinely offered, instead of the three recommended by NICE.

Ask your GP or contact your local CCG to find out what the criteria for NHS-funded IVF treatment are in your area.

Private treatment

If you're not eligible for NHS treatment or you decide to pay for IVF, you can have treatment at a private clinic. Some clinics can be contacted directly without seeing your GP first, but others may ask for a referral from your GP.

The cost of private treatment can vary, but one cycle of IVF can cost up to £5,000 or more. There may be additional costs for medicines, consultations and tests. During your discussions with the clinic, make sure you find out exactly what's included in the price.

Some people consider having IVF abroad, but there are a number of issues you need to think about, including your safety and the standard of care you'll receive. Clinics in other countries may not be as regulated as they are in the UK.

You can read about private fertility treatment and the issues and risks associated with fertility treatment abroad on the Human Fertilisation and Embryology Authority (HFEA) website.

1 June 2015

⇨ The above information is reprinted with kind permission from NHS Choices. Please visit www.nhs.uk for further information.

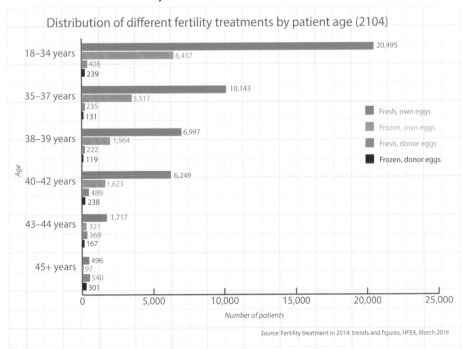

Distribution of different fertility treatments by patient age (2104)

Source: Fertility treatment in 2014: trends and figures, HFEA, March 2016

Scottish Government to fund three cycles of IVF

Minister says money has been "put aside" for programme, which follows National Infertility Group recommendations.

The Scottish Government is to fund three cycles of NHS IVF treatment for eligible couples trying to start a family – more than the number available in some parts of England and Wales.

Announcing the move, the public health minister, Aileen Campbell, defended the spending at a time of pressure on accident and emergency departments and waiting times.

Campbell told the BBC Radio 4 *Today* programme: "We have always had a commitment towards ensuring there is as equitable access to IVF as there possibly can be and we had a number of recommendations presented to us that we accepted from the National Infertility Group.

"One of these included ensuring that couples could get access to three cycles of IVF. That is today what we are taking forward.

"The very positive announcement of allowing couples who are desiring to have a family to get access to three cycles has been welcomed across the different fertility organisations."

The Scottish National Party minister said money had been "put aside" to fund the IVF programme.

Asked how she squared this with other demands on funding in the Scottish NHS, she said: "We have got a fairly strong record across Scotland on our NHS. Some of our A&Es have outperformed the lion's share of England's A&Es.

"We are outperforming A&Es across the UK and have done for some months. We have good investment levels in the NHS and we have record numbers of staff.

"We have got a commitment to our NHS that we will invest more money in our NHS than any of the other parties that stood in the election."

From 1 April, new patients referred for IVF treatment may be eligible for three full cycles rather than two, after the change was recommended to ministers by the National Infertility Group last year.

Campbell said: "We want to make access to treatment on the NHS as fair as possible – giving more people the opportunity to conceive. Over the last five years we have invested around £24 million to reduce IVF waiting times and improve the outcomes for couples. These changes make NHS IVF access in Scotland by far the fairest and most generous in the UK."

Scottish Labour's health spokesman, Anas Sarwar, said: "Scottish Labour argued in its manifesto for an increase in the number of full cycles of IVF available to couples from two to three. This is a very welcome and long-overdue announcement from the Scottish Government."

24 March 2017

⇨ The above information is reprinted with kind permission from the Press Association. Please visit www.pressassociation.com for further information.

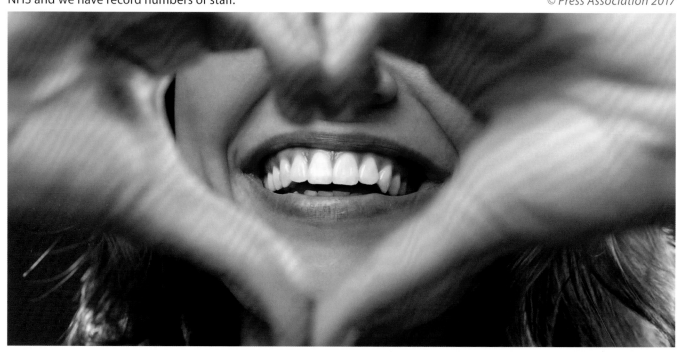

What is Clomid and how does it work? Fertility medication's side effects and success rate

It's commonly used for women with PCOS.

By Amy Packham

Women who suffer fertility problems will be offered different treatments depending on what's causing the problem.

However one of the most common fertility medicines on the NHS is clomifene, a medicine that encourages the monthly release of an egg in women who don't ovulate regularly or who can't at all.

Clomifene (which is often referred to by the brand name Clomid) is usually prescribed to women who have polycystic ovary syndrome (PCOS).

Using the fertility drug can also result in a greater chance of having twins.

We spoke to Dr Geeta Nargund, medical director of CREATE Fertility and Dr Kim Clugston, fertility expert at DuoFertility to find out more about the fertility treatment option.

How common is it for women to use Clomid?

Dr Nargund told HuffPost UK: "It is used in women with PCOS to induce ovulation and in those where ovulation is irregular to regularise ovulation.

"It is commonly used as an effective first-line treatment for ovulation induction and is widely available on NHS.

"However, it should be prescribed by a fertility specialist (not by a GP) after pre-treatment counselling and tests in order to ensure that the dosage is tailored to achieve successful outcome and avoid risks."

The most recent NICE guidelines suggest that Clomid should not be given to women with unexplained infertility as there is no evidence to suggest it increases pregnancy rates.

How does it work?

Women take one oral tablet daily (typically 50mg) for five consecutive days at the beginning of their cycle.

"Clomid is an anti-oestrogen," explained Dr Nargund. "It stimulates the pituitary gland to release hormones needed to stimulate ovulation."

Dr Clugston said it tricks the body into thinking that there is not enough oestrogen which sends a signal to the pituitary gland to secrete more follicle-stimulating hormone (FSH).

"This promotes the growth of follicles and the development of a usually a single dominant follicle that contains a mature egg which is released at ovulation," she said."

Are there any side effects of Clomid?

Clomid is generally "very well tolerated" explained Nargund.

"Mood swings are the most common side effect," she said. "Visual disturbances and hot flushes are rare side effects. Other rare side effects include pelvic discomfort, breast tenderness and nausea."

Ovarian Hyperstimulation Syndrome (OHSS) is a rare side effect that can result from an "over-response" to Clomid - this is a "rare but serious condition".

You should seek medical advice if these symptoms persist or become severe.

What's the success rate?

"The main aim of Clomid is to restore ovulation and it will do so in around 70-80% of women who take it," said Dr Clugston. "Once ovulating, these women have a chance of pregnancy, which is roughly 20% per cycle.

"Clomid is generally well tolerated by most women but it can have some negative effects on cervical mucus and on the endometrium, which may have an impact success rates. However, for women who are not ovulating naturally the benefit of ovulating outweighs these changes."

Women should talk to their GP regarding fertility treatment options. For more information on Clomid, visit the NHS Choices website.

30 March 2017

⇨ The above information is reprinted with kind permission from The Huffington Post UK. Please visit www.huffingtonpost.co.uk for further information.

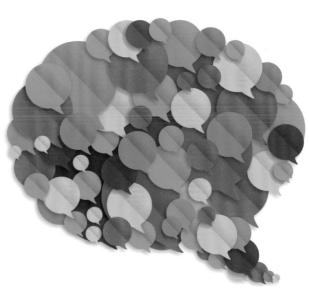

The advantages and disadvantages of IVF

Since IVF was pioneered by Sir Robert Edwards and Patrick Steptoe in 1978, IVF has helped thousands and thousands of people become parents. Here we outline some of the advantages and disadvantages associated with IVF. For more information, it is always best to see a fertility specialist who can advise you in more detail about IVF.

Advantages

IVF helps patients who would be otherwise unable to conceive. The ultimate advantage of IVF is achieving a successful pregnancy and a healthy baby. IVF can make this a reality for people who would be unable to have a baby otherwise.

Blocked tubes: For women with blocked or damaged fallopian tubes, IVF provides the best opportunity of having a child using their own eggs.

Older patients/patients with a low ovarian reserve: IVF can be used to maximise the chance of older patients conceiving. At CREATE, we have great expertise with older women and those with low ovarian reserve. We use Natural and Mild IVF to focus on quality of eggs, rather than quantity.

Male infertility: Couples with a male infertility problem will have a much higher chance of conceiving with IVF than conceiving naturally. We have a number of laboratory techniques to facilitate this including intra-cytoplasmic sperm injection (ICSI). We also liaise with an experienced urologist, Mr Vinod Nargund.

Unexplained infertility: one in six couples will suffer infertility problems and sometimes these remain undiagnosed after investigation. These patients may benefit from intervention.

PCOS: Polycystic ovary syndrome is a common condition in which there is a hormone imbalance leading to irregular menstrual cycles. IVF has proved very successful in patients with PCOS, who will not respond appropriately to fertility medication in isolation.

Endometriosis: Patients with endometriosis, where parts of the womb lining grow outside the womb, may like to try IVF, as it has proved successful in this group.

Premature ovarian failure: Women with premature ovarian failure or menopause can have IVF treatment using donor eggs, which typically has high success rates.

It has been used for a long time and has a safe track record. The first 'IVF baby', Louise Brown, was born using natural IVF in 1978. Since then, the technology has advanced, and techniques refined in order to create safe and successful treatment. We use only the safest forms of IVF with the lowest drug regimes in order to prevent side effects such as Ovarian Hyperstimulation Syndrome (OHSS).

IVF is more successful than IUI and other forms of assisted reproductive technology. IVF success rates have been increasing year on year since its conception, thanks to technological advances. Although IUI and other forms of assisted reproduction technology can be successful for some patients, on the whole they have not undergone the same level of improvement, and do not currently have as high success rates. IUI with donor sperm can however be a useful first option in single women and same-sex couples.

It can help single women and same-sex couples. For single women or same-sex couples who wish to have a child, IVF can provide a great opportunity for helping them to become parents. IVF with donor sperm can help potential patients achieve this goal.

It can help to diagnose fertilisation problems. In some cases of unexplained infertility, there could be a problem with fertilisation. Cases such as these may not be diagnosed until fertilisation is attempted in the laboratory. Although this would be a disappointing outcome, it is useful to be able to uncover such problems so that solutions can be reached for future treatment with ICSI.

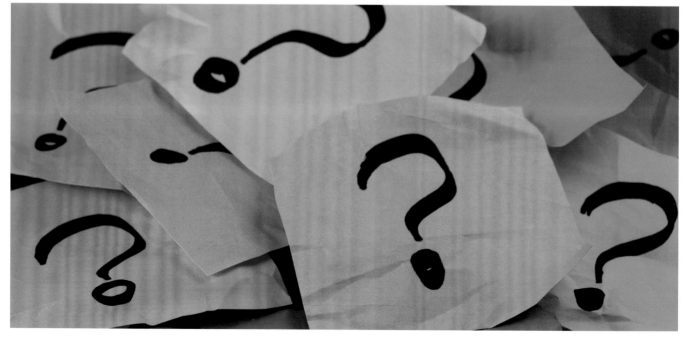

Unused embryos can be donated to research or another couple. If you are lucky enough to have embryos to spare, these can be used to help other people and even save lives. With the permission of the biological parents, unused embryos can be donated for research purposes, or to another couple to enable them to have a child.

It can be used to screen for inherited disease. For individuals who are known carriers of genetic disorders such as cystic fibrosis, Huntington's disease and muscular dystrophy, IVF with pre-implantation genetic diagnosis (PGD) is one of the most reliable ways to ensure that a child conceived will not suffer from the disorder. Pre-implantation genetic screening (PGS) can improve the chances of a successful cycle, as it screens embryos for chromosomal disorders such as Down's syndrome. Both of these techniques will shortly be available at our clinic.

Disadvantages

An IVF cycle may be unsuccessful. The success of IVF is not guaranteed, and patients often have to undergo more than one cycle of treatment before they are successful. Currently just over 25% of all IVF cycles result in a live birth. This naturally varies woman to woman, and a fertility specialist will be able to give a more accurate and personalised likelihood of success. It is important to be realistic but positive about the chances of success.

There may be associated side effects. As a medical treatment, IVF comes with a small chance of developing side effects, the most severe of these being severe ovarian hyper-stimulation syndrome (OHSS). Fortunately, the use of fewer or no drugs in natural and mild IVF cycles means that the already small likelihood of developing unwanted side effects is dramatically decreased or eliminated. CREATE Fertility takes the possibility of side effects very seriously, and as a result of our carefully constructed treatment protocols has never had a patient admitted to hospital with severe OHSS.

Multiple pregnancy. In IVF treatments, there is often more than one embryo put back into the uterus, and this leads to a higher likelihood of multiple pregnancy; around 20-30% of IVF pregnancies are multiple pregnancies. Multiple pregnancies do carry associated health risks to mother and baby: there is an increased chance of premature labour, miscarriage, need for caesarean, stillbirth and infant health problems with multiple pregnancies. It is important for all fertility clinics to have robust single embryo transfer policies, to avoid the risks of multiple pregnancy. At CREATE, we have a low multiple birth rate and focus on the reduction of multiple births.

There is a slightly higher chance of ectopic pregnancy. With IVF treatment, the risk of an ectopic pregnancy doubles, to 1–3%, particularly in women with damaged fallopian tubes.

There is evidence that high oestrogen levels associated with high stimulation IVF can cause prematurity of birth and low birth weight. There is growing evidence that giving high stimulation given to a woman during IVF increases the chance that a baby is born prematurely and with low birth weight. This has been linked to long-term health problems for the child. It is theorised that high oestrogen levels can affect the intra-uterine environment. With drug-free and low drug approaches, it has been observed that babies born are more likely to be born at full term and with a higher birth weight than those born through high stimulation IVF associated with high oestrogen levels. This is one of the reasons why we are committed to Natural and Mild IVF, as we believe that the success of treatment is not just a live birth, but is a healthy full term live birth.

IVF treatment can take an emotional/psychological toll. Going through IVF treatment can be a highly emotive and stressful experience. For patients undergoing treatment, it can be physically and emotionally demanding. For partners it can be difficult to watch a loved one go through a stressful experience. It is important to prioritise your psychological health, and this is also good for the health of the body. Our short, low-drug protocols should help to minimise the amount of stress.

IVF treatment can be expensive. IVF treatment is not cheap, and after paying for medication and blood tests, the costs can quickly mount up. It is good to have a clear idea of the costs involved before starting treatment, and to have your finances in order before beginning. With fewer drugs, the cost of a cycle is reduced at CREATE Fertility. There are also options for low-cost treatment, such as egg sharing and, in the future, our Walking Egg programme.

Some patients may be concerned about ethical issues. The idea of selecting some embryos and potentially discarding others may not sit well with everybody. Before starting treatment, consider your own stance and what you would be comfortable with. If you are uncomfortable with the creation of multiple embryos, we can support your choice by using Natural Cycle IVF, or by freezing additional eggs rather than fertilising them to create embryos.

⇨ The above information is reprinted with kind permission from CREATE Fertility. Please visit www.createhealth. org for further information.

©CREATE Fertility 2017

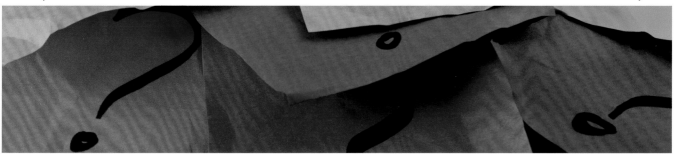

New 'IVF calculator' can predict couple's chance of conceiving baby, say experts

The tool, which can be used by doctors or people seeking fertility treatment, can estimate a couple's chance of having a baby before and after first IVF treatment, and over multiple cycles.

Writing in *The BMJ*, researchers led by the University of Aberdeen describe how the calculator could "help to shape couples' expectations".

It takes into account the age of a woman, how many years she has been trying to conceive, whether she has an ovulation problem, an unexplained fertility issue or whether there is a male fertility problem, among other factors.

The tool is based on data from the Human Fertilisation and Embryology Authority (HFEA), which collects information on all licensed fertility treatments in the UK.

The researchers analysed data from all women who started IVF and intracytoplasmic sperm injection (ICSI) in the UK from 1999 to 2008 using their own eggs and partner's sperm.

They found that of 114,000 women who completed almost 185,000 cycles of treatment, 29.1% had a live birth following their first cycle.

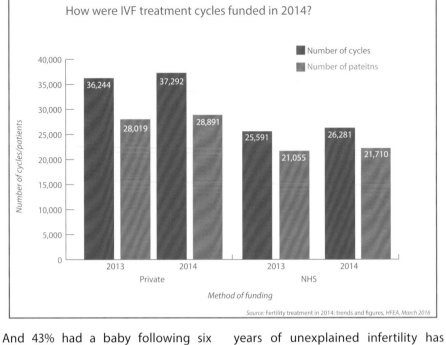

How were IVF treatment cycles funded in 2014?

Source: Fertility treatment in 2014: trends and figures, *HFEA, March 2016*

And 43% had a baby following six cycles of treatment.

They found that the chances of a couple having a baby declined after the woman reached the age of 30 and decreased with increasing duration of infertility.

The data was then put into the calculator to predict IVF success.

For example, the calculator predicts that a 30-year-old woman with two years of unexplained infertility has a 46% chance of having a live birth from the first complete cycle of IVF and a 79% chance over three complete cycles.

The calculator can be found at w3.abdn.ac.uk/clsm/opis.

Professor Adam Balen, chairman of the British Fertility Society, said: "This is an important paper which analyses the HFEA database to calculate prediction models for success based upon baseline characteristics and the data collected during the treatment.

"The database is huge and so the information gathered is clinically relevant.

"It is important to remember that treatment should be individualised to the patients' particular needs and profile and it can still be difficult to accurately predict the outcome."

16 November 2016

⇨ The above information is reprinted with kind permission from the Press Association. Please visit www.pressassociation.com for further information.

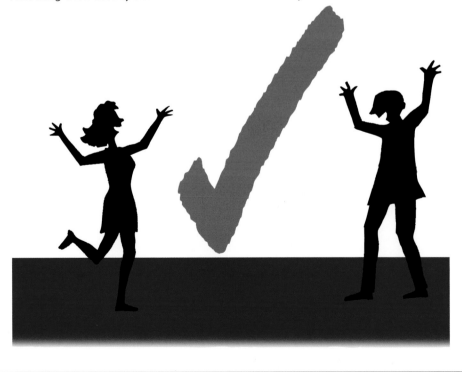

IVF has little effect on health of the child

An article from The Conversation.

THE CONVERSATION

By Jordana Bell, Senior Lecturer, King's College London, Jeffrey Craig, Principal Research Fellow, Murdoch Childrens Research Institute and Juan Castillo-Fernandez, PhD candidate, King's College London

The rate of IVF births has risen dramatically in recent years as fertility rates continue to fall worldwide. To date, over five million babies have been born with the help of these technologies. However, there have been concerns about potential health problems in children conceived by IVF. Our latest study shows that those fears are largely unfounded.

Since the first IVF baby was born in 1978, scientists have raised concerns about potential birth defects and health problems in children conceived by IVF. Most of the children appear healthy, but a small increase in health problems, such as low birth weight, premature birth and birth defects, has been reported. Since IVF has only been available for about 40 years, the long-term health effects of this technology have not yet been fully explored.

There is growing evidence that certain risk factors, such as poor maternal nutrition, at the time of conception and pregnancy can influence a person's health in later life. Recent studies have shown that some of these long-term health effects may be encoded by epigenetics.

Epigenetics are the biological mechanisms that regulate genes. Epigenetic switches control whether genes are activated or silenced. Events that occur in early development, including the time between conception and birth, can influence health in later life and epigenetics play an important role in this process.

Previous research has studied the link between epigenetics and IVF, but the results have been inconsistent. One reason for this is that fertility treatment is often associated with common risk factors, aside from the IVF technology itself, such as being older mums or having twins or triplets, which are more likely to be delivered prematurely and have a lower birth weight.

The twin approach

In our study, we examined epigenetic changes in IVF and naturally conceived newborn twins. We only considered babies born from twin pregnancies to avoid finding epigenetic differences attributed to single and multiple births.

Most of the previous epigenetic studies in IVF focused on selected regions of the genome that regulate genes known to cause developmental disorders due to epigenetic alterations, but we investigated the entire genome to ask if there were differences in genes that had not been previously implicated in epigenetic disorders.

We found no major epigenetic differences in IVF-conceived twins, but we did find epigenetic changes with small impacts. Two genes related to male and female infertility showed small but significant differences in IVF-conceived twins, which suggests that the newborn twin epigenetic profile may contain markers of parental infertility, to a small extent. But it is unclear if the small changes that we saw were a result of infertility or the IVF treatment itself.

Twins provide a natural unique study design that allows us to separate the importance of genes and environment on human traits. Environment exposures can be shared by both twins in a pair, for example in the womb, or exposures can also be specific to each twin. Using this twin-based approach we found that environmental factors specific to each twin were most likely to influence the top IVF-associated epigenetic changes. One explanation for these results could be that the IVF procedure introduces slight variability in epigenetic marks.

Epigenetic differences have been identified in common chronic diseases such as cancer, psychiatric disorders and diabetes. We found no such major epigenetic differences in babies conceived by IVF, although future studies are needed to see if the small epigenetic changes we observed remain over time. Our results are reassuring for parents who used IVF and children conceived by IVF as our research suggests that IVF technology has little impact on epigenetic changes, and potentially future health.

28 March 2017

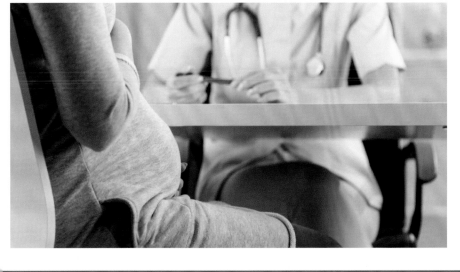

Does IVF cut birth defect risk in babies with older mothers?

" Women aged 40 or over are less likely to have babies with birth defects if they conceive by IVF," the Daily Mail reports, while the *Daily Telegraph* says: "Older mothers have healthier babies if they conceive using IVF."

Both headlines misinterpret the results of a study that looked at births in South Australia between 14 and 30 years ago.

Researchers wanted to see which maternal factors were linked to the risk of birth defects, and how this risk compared between women who conceived naturally and those who had two types of fertility treatment: either in vitro fertilisation (IVF) or intracytoplasmic sperm injection (ICSI).

Overall, they found there were three lifestyle factors linked to birth defects: maternal age, whether the mother was a smoker and how many children she'd had before.

Among the smaller proportion of women who had IVF or ICSI, increasing age was not linked with birth defects with either of these individual fertility methods. However, when the researchers combined the two groups they found reduced risk of birth defects for women over 40.

However, this finding does not prove that fertility treatment is definitely 'safer' in older women and more likely to result in a healthy baby. These analyses involve smaller numbers of women and babies. There is also likely to be a complex interplay between a wide range of factors and the risk of birth defects.

You can reduce the risk of pregnancy complications by taking the recommended vitamin D and folic acid supplements and avoiding smoking, drinking alcohol and taking illegal drugs.

Where did the story come from?

The study was carried out by researchers from the University of Adelaide and the University of Melbourne.

It was funded by the National Health and Medical Research Council and the Australian Research Council.

The study was published in the peer-reviewed *British Journal of Obstetrics and Gynaecology*.

Both the *Mail* and the *Telegraph's* reporting may give a confusing message to older women planning a pregnancy that fertility treatment is the safer way to conceive a healthy baby after the age of 40.

The media do not present the full nature of the links and also grouped their reporting to talk of IVF being linked to reduced risk. In fact IVF was not linked with increased age at all – neither an increased or decreased risk – it was only when pooling with ICSI that a significant result was found.

What kind of research was this?

This retrospective cohort study aimed to look at the maternal factors associated with birth defects in women who either conceived naturally

or had two different types of fertility treatment: IVF or ICSI.

IVF and ICSI are both assisted reproduction techniques. In IVF, an egg is incubated in the laboratory with many sperm, while in ICSI a single sperm is directly injected into the egg.

ICSI may be used when there are problems with the sperm that may limit the chances of conception happening 'naturally' in IVF – for example, problems with how well the sperm can 'swim' towards the egg.

A cohort study can look at the links between particular maternal factors, the conception method and the chances of a birth defect.

But it's likely there is a complex interaction of confounding factors associated with all these issues, meaning one has not necessarily caused the other.

What did the research involve?

The study reviewed all assisted reproduction technologies carried out in South Australia over a 16-year period from 1986 to 2002.

This was linked to data on birth outcomes from the South Australian Birth Defects Register (SABDR). The register includes a record of all live births, stillbirths, terminations, birth weight and congenital defects. Birth defects were also followed up for five years.

Maternal medical conditions, pre-existing and pregnancy-related, were reviewed in the women's medical records.

The researchers looked at the statistical link between maternal factors and birth defects, and compared this between babies either conceived naturally or by IVF and ICSI.

What were the basic results?

There were 2,211 IVF births, 1,399 ICSI births and 301,060 naturally conceived births during the study period.

There were double the proportion of women aged 40 or over in the IVF

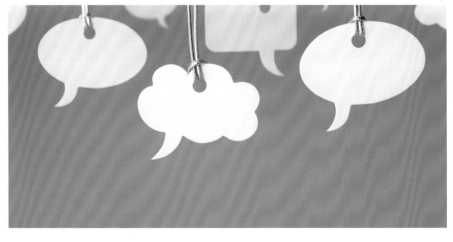

(112, 5.1%) and ICSI (63, 4.5%) groups compared with the natural conception group (4,992, 1.7%).

The prevalence of any birth defects was 7.1% (157) in the IVF group, 9.9% (138) in the ICSI group and 5.8% (17,408) in the natural conception group.

The researchers found several factors were associated with an increased risk of birth defects in each of the groups, including three lifestyle factors.

Age

Compared with women aged 30 to 34:

⇨ natural conception group: age above 35 increased risk, age below 30 decreased risk

⇨ IVF group: age below 30 increased risk, but no link for age above 35

⇨ ICSI group: no link with any age

⇨ However, pooling the IVF and ICSI groups found an increased risk for women below 30 and a decreased risk for women above 40"

Number of previous children or births

Compared with one previous birth:

⇨ natural conception group: increased risk with first birth, decreased risk for two or more prior births

⇨ IVF group: no link

⇨ ICSI: increased risk with first birth, no link for two or more births.

Smoking

⇨ natural conception group: increased risk

⇨ IVF and ICSI: no link.

How did the researchers interpret the results?

The researchers concluded: "The usual age–birth defect relationship is reversed in births after IVF and ICSI, and the associations for other maternal factors and defects vary between IVF and ICSI."

Conclusion

The media has rather a simplistic take on this retrospective cohort study. The study has not proven that women are more likely to have a healthier baby if they have IVF if they are over the age of 40.

The misguided headlines may prompt some women aged 40 or over to think they should seek fertility treatment to give them the best chance of having a healthy baby.

But, regardless of your age, there is no reason to consider fertility treatment if you are able to conceive naturally.

Despite the large cohort included in this study, some of the analyses only looked at small numbers – for example, the number of birth defects was small, and there was only a small number of women aged over 40 relative to the whole population.

This means it's possible that some of the links found may be down to chance, particularly as the study did not set out to explore the link with any specific factor.

Also, having IVF over the age of 40 didn't decrease the risk of birth defects, as the media has implied – there was no significant link with increased age in the IVF group. It was only when pooling with the ICSI group that a statistical link was found.

The study also looked at data from between 14 and 30 years ago in Australia. This may not be relevant to either women in the UK or current lifestyles and medical care.

There is likely to be a complex interaction between different factors associated with the age a women has a baby, the conception method and reasons for this choice, and the risk of birth defects.

Despite careful adjustment for confounding, in a population-level observational study it is always going to be difficult to fully account for all factors.

Paternal factors are one notable exception that haven't been considered. As such, there is a high chance that confounding factors have influenced any of the links found.

Overall, the findings of this study should not be of concern to women aged over 40, many of whom go on to have healthy pregnancies without the need for fertility treatment.

Analysis by Bazian. Edited by NHS Choices. Follow NHS Choices on Twitter. Join the Healthy Evidence forum.

17 October 2016

⇨ The above information is reprinted with kind permission from NHS Choices. Please visit www.nhs.uk for further information.

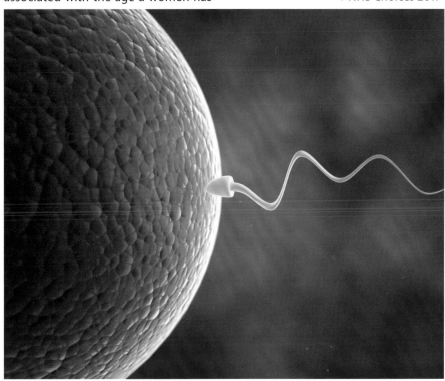

Surrogacy in the UK: myth busting and reform

Report of the Surrogacy UK Working Group on Surrogacy Law.

Surrogacy in the UK: setting the scene

Surrogacy arrangements have been regulated in the UK since 1985. The Surrogacy Arrangements Act 1985 reflected the state of knowledge and societal beliefs about surrogacy at the time and was largely based on recommendations made in the Warnock Report. Though some further regulation of aspects of surrogacy (most notably how legal parenthood can be transferred to the intended parents (IPs) from the surrogate and her partner) occurred in primary legislation in both the 1990 and 2008 Human Fertilisation and Embryology (HFE) Acts, as well as in some other pieces of secondary legislation, the law pertaining to surrogacy is now 30 years old and increasingly out of date. It does not reflect the realities of modern surrogacy and needs thorough review by lawmakers, with a view to bringing the law in line with the views and needs of the families – and reflecting the best interests of the children – created by this method.

The time since the Surrogacy Arrangements Act has seen major social change: not least the birth of the Internet and cheap, easy overseas travel for fertility treatment (often dubbed "reproductive tourism"), but also changes in the types and variety of family form (and ways of forming families) that have come to be accepted. There have also been significant legal changes, including the passage of the Human Rights Act 1998 as well as the introduction of, first, civil partnerships and, more recently, same-sex marriage in 2014. Additionally, burgeoning surrogacy markets have emerged in various countries, notably parts of the US, India, Thailand or Nepal – or are beginning to emerge (e.g. Mexico, Cambodia, Greece).

Reliable data on the number of surrogacy arrangements being entered into by parents from the UK, whether domestic or overseas arrangements, is notoriously hard to obtain, as has been remarked upon by numerous academic commentators over many years. This is not helped by the fact that different government agencies record different aspects of the process, using different timelines and parameters. It is also probably the case that some families created by surrogacy are not recorded at all, particularly if there is no clinical involvement in their creation. In addition, despite the findings and recommendations of the Brazier Report in 1998, little has changed in terms of surrogacy's regulation. In fact, it is an enduring truth that "the law governing surrogacy remains confused, incoherent, and poorly adapted to the specific realities of the practice of surrogacy". On a positive note, however, an ongoing longitudinal study has shown that the psychological well-being of children born and families created through surrogacy in the UK is not in question, and there have been published studies showing that motivations and experiences of women who become surrogates are generally positive.

This working group started from the premise that so much information on surrogacy arrangements is missing from public, political, legal and social discourse – particularly what kinds of arrangement (domestic or overseas, altruistic or commercial, etc.) are entered into by Intended Parents (IPs) from the UK, and how people experience them. Rather, what have come into existence, and seem to persist, are a series of 'surrogacy myths', which have influenced policy and debate to date. As part of our work towards this report, we commissioned our own survey on people's views of surrogacy practices and the law that relates to surrogacy, with a view to interrogating some of these surrogacy myths and finding out what really happens in surrogacy arrangements in the UK. We received an unprecedented number of responses, particularly from within the surrogacy community (surrogates and IPs).

Key findings:

⇨ Reliable data on surrogacy in the UK is largely absent, including that relating to the number of IPs travelling overseas for surrogacy.

⇨ As a result of the lack of good data, a number of 'surrogacy myths' have been born, which have informed much of the public, political, legal and social debate on surrogacy.

For references, see full report.

November 2015

⇨ The above information is reprinted with kind permission from Surrogacy UK. Please visit www.surrogacyuk.org for further information.

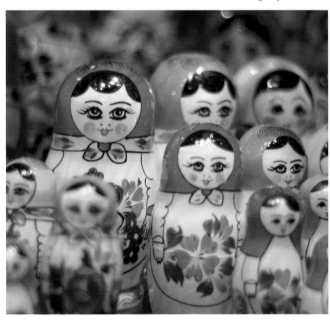

Surrogacy: legal rights of parents and surrogates

1. Overview

If you use a surrogate they will be the legal mother of any child they carry.

Mother's rights

The woman who gives birth is always treated as the mother in UK law and has the right to keep the child – even if they're not genetically related. However, parenthood can be transferred by parental order or adoption.

Surrogacy contracts aren't enforced by UK law, even if you've signed a deal with your surrogate and have paid for her expenses.

It's illegal to pay a surrogate in the UK, except for their reasonable expenses.

Father's rights

The child's legal father or 'second parent' will be the surrogate's husband or partner unless:

⇨ legal rights are given to someone else through a parental order or adoption

⇨ the surrogate's husband or civil partner didn't give their permission to their wife or partner.

If your surrogate has no partner, or they're unmarried and not in a civil partnership, the child will have no legal father or second parent unless the partner actively consents.

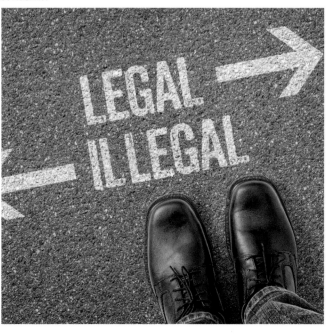

2. Become the child's legal parent

You must apply for a parental order if you want to become the legal parent of the child.

Parental orders

You must be genetically related to a child to apply for a parental order, i.e. the egg or sperm donor, and in a relationship where you and your partner are either:

⇨ married

⇨ civil partners

⇨ living as partners

⇨ You and your partner must also:

⇨ have the child living with you

⇨ reside permanently in either the UK, Channel Islands or Isle of Man.

You can't apply for a parental order if you're single.

How to apply

You must fill in a C51 application form for a parental order and give this to a family proceedings court within 6 months of the child's birth.

You don't have to use your local family proceedings court, but you'll need to explain why not if you don't.

You'll need to provide the child's full birth certificate and will also be charged a court fee of £200.

The court will then set a date for the hearing and issue you with a C52 acknowledgement form that you must give to the child's legal parent, i.e. your surrogate.

The birth mother and anyone else who's a parent of the child must agree to the parental order in writing.

You can't apply for a parental order once the child is older than six months.

Adoption

If neither you or your partner are related to the child, or you're single, adoption is the only way you can become the child's legal parent.

Donor's rights

If you use donated sperm or eggs with your surrogate, read about the rights of your donor.

3. Children born outside the UK

If your surrogate gives birth abroad, you can only apply for a parental order if you and your partner are living in the UK.

The child will need a visa to enter the UK during this process.

Using a surrogate abroad can be complicated because different countries have different rules. You may want to get legal advice or contact the The Human Fertilisation and Embryology Authority for more information.

4. Pay and leave

You and your partner may be eligible for adoption pay and leave and paternity pay and leave if you use a surrogate.

If you're not eligible for paid leave, you may be able to take parental leave or annual leave.

Surrogates

Every pregnant employee has the right to 52 weeks' maternity leave and to return to their job after this.

What a birth mother does after the child is born has no impact on her right to maternity leave.

⇨ The above information is reprinted with kind permission from GOV. UK. Please visit GOV.UK for further information.

British public: legalise paid surrogacy

Most people in Britain approve of paid surrogate pregnancies – but public support is lower when it is used by gay couples.

Recently an Australian couple were accused of abandoning a child with Down's syndrome and a heart condition with his surrogate mother in Thailand, while taking home to Australia the child's healthy twin sister. The details of the case are murky – the surrogacy agent who arranged the deal claims the couple later offered to take the child – but the incident shed light on the issue of regulation in surrogacy.

Surrogacy itself, or the process of a 'surrogate' mother carrying a child for someone else, has been regulated under British law since the 1980s. In 1985, the Surrogacy Arrangements Act made commercial surrogacy – when the surrogate is paid a fee – prohibited, so surrogates in the UK must currently be volunteers (though they can be paid for reasonable expenses related to the surrogacy).

New YouGov research finds that the law is out of sync with British public opinion on this issue.

59% of British adults now approve of the process called 'gestational' surrogacy: when a woman carries another couple's fertilised embryo in her womb from pregnancy to birth, even though she has no biological connection to the child. 21% disapprove people using this process to have children.

By a slightly narrower margin, 54% to 26%, the British public also support making it legal to pay a surrogate. In both cases, support is higher among younger adults, although people who are positive about surrogacy outweigh the detractors across all age groups.

There is no ban on commercial surrogacy in the United States, at least on the federal level, and states like California and Illinois both permit and facilitate surrogacy arrangements. Other states do not recognise these arrangements or prohibit them.

By 69% to 16%, Americans approve of couples using gestational surrogacy, and by a near-identical margin (69% to 15%) say it should be legal to pay a surrogate.

Surrogacy and sexual orientation

A recent headline in the *Daily Mail* newspaper caused controversy when it described a proposed NHS sperm bank – a key resource for some couples when pursuing surrogacy – as "for lesbians", though it technically made its services available to all women and couples, gay or straight.

The incident underscores how social sensitivities can complicate the debate over processes like IVF and surrogacy.

Indeed, YouGov's research finds that there is lower support for surrogacy when it involves a gay couple seeking a surrogate rather than a heterosexual couple. In fact, telling respondents the couple using surrogacy is gay lowers approval of the process much more than telling respondents the couple is paying their surrogate.

To test this, YouGov asked half of respondents two questions about a 'married gay male couple' using surrogacy – one question asked about the use of a paid surrogate and one asked about a volunteer surrogate. The other half of respondents were asked the same two questions, but about a "married heterosexual couple".

When the couple is straight, most British people approve of the surrogacy arrangement, whether it is paid or voluntary (though support is eight points lower for the paid arrangement). When the couple is gay, support falls around 15 points for both arrangements.

Here, the age of the respondent becomes much more consequential: Adults over 40 tend to approve of the straight arrangements and tend to disapprove of the gay arrangements. On the other hand, by wide margins, under-40s approve of the surrogacy arrangements in all four scenarios, with only slightly lower approval in the case of the gay couple.

In the United States, the overall effect is even more dramatic: Americans are more approving than British people when it comes to the heterosexual couple, and divided on the gay couple in proportions virtually identical to those found in Britain.

8 August 2014

⇨ The above information is reprinted with kind permission from YouGov. Please visit www.yougov.co.uk for further information.

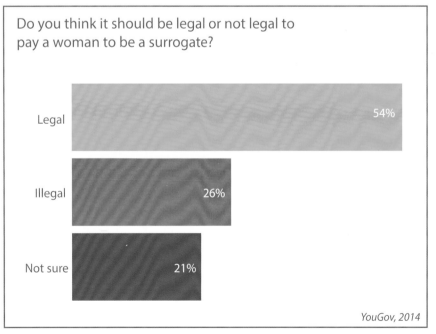

Do you think it should be legal or not legal to pay a woman to be a surrogate?

- Legal — 54%
- Illegal — 26%
- Not sure — 21%

YouGov, 2014

Fostering and adoption

What's involved and what you need to do.

Giving vulnerable children a safe environment

If you've decided you want to help vulnerable children – giving them a loving, stable home while local authorities find a long-term place for them, it's worth finding out more about fostering. When you plan to adopt, it can also help if you look after vulnerable children as early as possible, before adopting them permanently. Here we explain the various options and what's involved.

Considering fostering?

Foster care is quite different from adoption, giving children loving, stable care until they can return to their own family or move on elsewhere. There are over 44,000 children and young people in foster care throughout the UK, and there's a major shortage of foster carers. So if you want to give vulnerable children a loving, stable environment while authorities find a healthy long-term solution for them, fostering could be for you.

Fostering for adoption

You might also want to consider fostering, so you can start looking after children you hope to adopt. Fostering for adoption is a quite recent initiative, designed to get children into a permanent, loving home as early as possible, with a view to adoption further down the line. It's aimed at people who have been approved both as foster carers and for adoption – this means children can be placed with you on a temporary basis, so if the court later agrees that the child should be adopted, the placement moves from fostering to adoption. For a child who craves stability, this option means they can be adopted with minimum disruption.

Adopting

When you adopt, you're providing a new, permanent family for children who can no longer live with their own family. Adoption is the best option for a minority of children, with around 4,000 children needing adoptive families each year.

Find out more

All these options can be wonderful for children who need love and care, and for parents who really want to build a family. It's a major decision to take and there's a lot of information and advice to help you decide whether fostering and adoption are for you.

The British Association for Adoption & Fostering (BAAF) – for advice on all aspects of adoption

NHS Choices – for an overview of the issues and options

Can I adopt?

The good news is anyone aged 21 or above can adopt – single, married, in a civil partnership or living with a partner. You don't have to own your own home and you don't have to be in work – what matters the most is giving the child a loving, happy family.

What does adoption involve?

Children who are available for adoption are usually being looked after by a local authority. So you'll need to apply to an adoption agency, who will need to approve you as suitable adoptive parents, match you with a child (or children) and support you through the whole adoption process.

Because it's so important to get it right, adoption agencies do everything they can to make adoptions work. This means the process can be pretty lengthy and demanding. You'll need to have medical checks, in-depth interviews with a social worker, police checks and home visits. It might feel intrusive at the time, but it's all in the interests of getting it right.

Are you right for adoption?

Do you have what it takes to be an adoptive parent? We hear from the Blackpool Council Adoption Services team around the traits which they deem to be fundamental in prospective adoptive parents...

Flexibility

In the UK, up to 39 weeks' statutory adoption pay is available to eligible

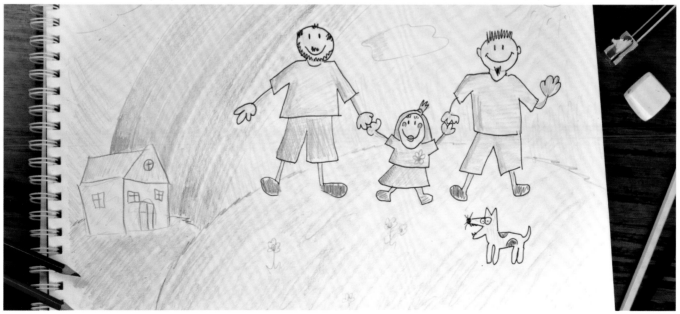

employees. An employee who is entitled to adoption leave can take up to 26 weeks' ordinary adoption leave, followed by a further 26 weeks of additional adoption leave.

Adoptive parents need to be flexible in terms of work to have the necessary quality time to bond and form a strong relationship.

Calming and understanding

A good listening ear is a must. We always look for people who are willing to learn and seek support but that are willing to give their new adoptive child the physical and emotional support they need.

Kindness

Being kind is fundamentally crucial. It's important to be as approachable and honest as possible and provide reassurance as the child's new forever family.

Recognition and awareness

It can be extremely helpful to allow your child to have a good understanding and awareness of their identity and background. We encourage the use of a life story book, which explains their history in an appropriate way as a means of them learning and becoming comfortable with their history and subsequent adoption journey.

Their past will always have an impact on their present and their future; however, by recognising this and bearing it in mind, whilst being open and approachable, can help both parents and children move forward.

Do I need special skills for different types of adoption?

As mentioned above, there are certain skills which we look for in candidates who want to adopt. There are, however, certain types of cases or times in a child's life that are special and require slightly more consideration.

Teens

One of the most underlying issues with adopted children when reaching their teenage years is helping them to understand their identity. All teenagers struggle with the concept of "Who am I?" and "What is my purpose?" but this can be extremely hard to understand and answer as the questions adoptive teens face are more complex than their non-adopted peers.

Give your teenager the information they need, help them learn more and be there to support them through the process.

Give them a voice in decisions, independence and most importantly, talk openly about issues.

Babies

Adoptive parents need to have the same qualities as any other new parent. It is a lifelong commitment that will bring out many sleepless nights, feeds and nappy changes.

The bond between you and the baby can take a little time to develop, so be patient and reassured that this is completely normal.

Children with disabilities

It's crucial that a prospective parent who wants to adopt a child with learning or physical disabilities is fully aware and able to cater to their needs.

Alternative approaches to communication may be required and additional skills may be needed for intellectual, sensory or other impairments.

You don't necessarily have to have experience with disabled children as long as you can demonstrate interest, commitment and willingness to care whilst undertaking research on the issues that need to be considered.

What are the first steps if I want to adopt?

The first thing to do is to contact your local adoption agency – visit the British Association for Adoption and Fostering (BAAF), or your local authority at the DirectGov website.

You can then read all about adoption, chat to people who have already adopted and have some counselling to help you understand the needs of children who may have been neglected or abused. Then, if you and the agency are still keen to go ahead, you can start applying!

What support is there for adoptive parents?

You'll get advice, information and counselling for adoptive parents from your local authority. Charities like Adoption UK and BAAF offer support too.

Getting the timing right

Everyone is different, but some people who haven't been able to conceive feel real grief and loss, so it's a good idea to come to terms with your situation before getting ready to move on and embrace a different kind of parenting.

For this reason, most adoption agencies ask you to wait several months after ending fertility treatment before you apply for approval. This gives you time to read up on adoption issues, chat to other people who are adopting, and hang out with kids to help you prepare!

Caring for your adopted child

Many of the children adopted from care will have experienced trauma and loss, even if they were adopted shortly after birth. Some may have additional needs resulting from physical, mental or emotional problems or disabilities. So it makes sense to talk to your partner, close friends and family about your thoughts and feelings, helping you prepare for the adoption process itself and also for coping better when you have children placed with you.

Finding a match

It's an exciting and emotional time when a possible match is suggested for you and a child. You need to find out as much as possible about the child's health history and needs, so you decide to go ahead you will be as well informed as possible. Having realistic expectations will increase the chances of the adoption working well.

⇨ The above information is reprinted with kind permission from Bounty. Please visit www.bounty.com for further information.

Woman gives birth to baby after having ovary tissue removed and frozen as a child in 'world first'

"This is a ground-breaking step."

By Amy Packham

A woman has given birth using frozen ovarian tissue that was removed when she was a child.

Moaza Al Matrooshi, 24, is thought to be the first person "in the world" to deliver a baby after having an ovary removed and frozen before she went through puberty.

Al Matrooshi, originally from Dubai, was eight when she had the organ removed before undergoing chemotherapy and a bone marrow transplant for her inherited blood disorder Beta Thalassaemia.

Her remaining ovary was only partially functioning following the chemotherapy and she went into early menopause. As she had not entered puberty, she could not have IVF treatment to allow her ovaries to produce eggs.

"Moaza has become the first woman in the world to give birth following the transplant of her own ovarian tissue removed before puberty," Rob Smith, clinic director at CARE London, the fertility centre where Al Matrooshi was treated, told PA.

Doctors transplanted the frozen ovarian tissue back into Al Matrooshi when she was 21 to give her a chance of conceiving using her own eggs.

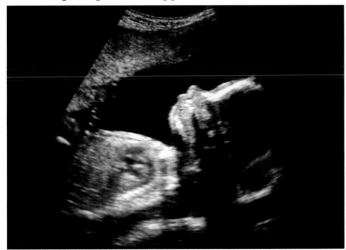

The new mum then underwent IVF treatment at CARE Fertility with her partner Ahmed and she gave birth to a baby boy on Tuesday 13 December.

Smith said the birth represented a "landmark in fertility preservation treatment for young girls who risk irreversible ovarian damage following necessary treatments for diseases such as cancer".

He said Al Matrooshi's story was a "beacon of hope to all women who face the prospect of infertility due to invasive treatments at a young age" and sent his "warmest congratulations" to the new family.

"We believe this case is an incredible example of how far IVF has come," he added.

"In the 15 years since Moaza's ovary was frozen, the success rates for IVF have improved dramatically allowing her to have an excellent chance of achieving a successful pregnancy."

Professor Adam Balen, chair of the British Fertility Society, said, according to PA: "This is a ground-breaking step in this area of fertility preservation and has the potential to help many young people who face cancer treatment preserve their fertility chances in the future.

"Storing ovarian tissue was pioneered 20 years ago and now the results are coming through. Chemotherapy and radiotherapy can have serious side effects on the reproductive organs.

"Storing ovarian tissue and more recently storing testicular tissue is becoming more mainstream, but we need more centres providing this service and it is important that a multi-disciplinary team of experts is involved to ensure young people in particular are offered this as an option."

15 December 2016

⇨ The above information is reprinted with kind permission from The Huffington Post UK. Please visit www.huffingtonpost.co.uk for further information.

Artificial eggs from stem cells marks fertility breakthrough – but human application is a long way off

Mouse pups born through technique were normal with no sign of premature death.

By Adam Watkins

Scientists have for the first time shown that fully mature egg cells can be grown in the lab, raising hope for new infertility treatments.

Until now, researchers have only been able to produce cells that resemble sperm or eggs, but which can rarely produce live offspring because of abnormal organisation of their genetic material. But a team at Kyushu University, Japan, have now turned stem cells from mice into mature eggs that can be fertilised and develop into healthy, fertile adults. This could lead to a way for women who can't naturally produce working eggs to have new ones made from their own cells.

Embryonic stem cells are living cells taken from an embryo that have the ability to develop into any other kind of cell. The researchers from the Kyushu University team previously demonstrated that, under the right conditions, these cells could be turned into primordial germ cells, immature embryonic versions of sperm and eggs. But because they are immature, these germ cells can't produce any offspring.

So the researchers adapted their methods to encase the stem cells in other cells taken from a mouse's foetal gonad (the developing ovary or testis). This recreated an environment more like an ovary and, over a period of four to five weeks, the team saw the stem cells develop into cells resembling mature eggs.

Functioning egg cells

While the cells looked like mature eggs, the key question was whether they actually were functional egg cells. The team compared their lab-grown eggs with ones from an ovary and found they were the same size and organised their genetic material in similar patterns.

The researchers also showed that their eggs could be fertilised, implanted into a surrogate female and go on to produce live offspring. But only a very small number of their embryos created in this way developed fully to term – just 3.5% of all the embryos they transferred. Importantly though, the team reported that "all the obtained pups grew up normally without evidence of premature death".

As all good scientists should, the researchers then replicated their experiments to test how robust their technique was. Initially, they used embryonic stem cells in their experiments, but these create an ethical dilemma because an embryo has to be destroyed to produce them.

In 2006, however, another researcher named Shinya Yamanaka and his team found that turning on just four specific genes in normal adult cells gives them all the potential to develop into other cells just like embryonic stem cells, but without the need to destroy a single embryo. The latest research showed that eggs made from these 'induced pluripotent stem cells', or IPSCs, were just as capable of being fertilised and producing healthy adult offspring as embryonic stem cells.

Research challenges

The findings from this study have clear implications for the treatment of human infertility. Being able to manufacture working eggs from regular cells could allow doctors to provide an alternative for women who don't naturally produce functional eggs. But, as with all research studies like this, there are still some limitations that need to be addressed.

First, the overall success rate of this technique is still low – just 3.5% of all embryos implanted gave rise to live offspring, compared to 30% of those currently used for human IVF treatment. Obviously, this would need to be improved, potentially by using different lab conditions, hormonal treatments or by encasing the stem cells in adult gonadal cells rather than foetal ones. However, improving the efficiency of such complex lab techniques can be very difficult.

Second, this study was conducted in mice and not humans. While the two species are similar in the way their eggs and embryos develop, there are some key differences. So scientists still need to prove they can replicate the technique with human cells.

Finally, while the researchers went to great lengths to show that the eggs, embryos and offspring generated in this study were "normal", the lab-grown eggs did display altered genetic patterns and unusual placenta growth. This means we need to research the full impact of the techniques used in this study on the long-term health of any offspring generated.

Still, the findings from this study open up new possibilities for the preservation and even restoration of fertility in women. As always these kinds of scientific breakthroughs, while there are clear benefits for many people, they also carry potential ethical implications. But the team at Kyushu University have pushed the boundaries of reproductive biology, opening new avenues that may one day help millions.

12 January 2017

⇨ The above information is reprinted with kind permission from *IB Times*. Please visit www.ibtimes.co.uk for further information.

Mitochondrial donation

Mitochondrial donation is an IVF technique that gives families affected by mitochondrial disease the chance of having healthy children.

It involves taking the DNA out of a woman's egg that has faulty mitochondria (the 'batteries' that give all our cells their energy), and transferring it to a donor egg with healthy mitochondria.

Our position

We actively support mitochondrial donation and have driven legislative change to ensure this cutting-edge technique can be used in clinics for the benefit of patients.

As a result of our work, and the work of others, the UK Parliament voted in support of mitochondrial donation in February 2015.

Since October 2015, mitochondrial donation has been licensed and regulated by the Human Fertilisation and Embryology Authority for clinical use in the UK.

What we're doing

Why does mitochondrial donation matter?

Approximately one in 200 children in the UK are born with faulty mitochondrial DNA.

While many people have mild or no symptoms, around one in 6,500 may develop more serious mitochondrial disorders.

In many families, mitochondrial disease affects multiple family members.

The disease can occur at a young age and lead to disability and death. Currently there is no cure.

Exploring the policy issues

For more than a decade, we've worked to engage with the public, parliamentarians and others about mitochondrial disease and donation.

We've provided opportunities for people to explore the techniques and their implications through events and communications.

Our partners have included biomedical and social scientists, ethicists and biomedical research and patient charities.

Providing long-term funding

We've provided long-term funding to establish and support researchers at the Wellcome Trust Centre for Mitochondrial Research at Newcastle University who pioneered the donation technique.

We'll continue to consider applications for research funding related to these technologies.

Timeline of key dates

Our timeline sets out the key dates which led to the licensing of mitochondrial donation.

2000

The Chief Medical Officers's expert group report, *Stem Cell Research: Medical Progress with Responsibility*, recognises the future potential use of mitochondrial donation.

2005

Researchers at Newcastle University obtain a research licence to work with human oocytes to explore mitochondrial donation techniques.

The House of Commons Science and Technology Committee publishes an extensive report, *Human Reproductive Technologies and the Law*, which supports further research in the area.

2008

The Government passes The Human Fertilisation and Embryology Act 2008, allowing researchers to develop techniques to prevent transmission of maternally inherited mitochondrial disease.

2010

Researchers at Newcastle University develop mitochondrial donation techniques to prevent diseased mitochondria being passed from mother to child.

2011

The Human Fertilisation and Embryology Authority convenes an Expert Scientific Review panel to assess the effectiveness and safety of mitochondrial donation.

May 2012

The Wellcome Centre for Mitochondrial Research (opens in a new tab), based at Newcastle University, is established with the aim of developing a programme of basic and clinical mitochondrial disease research.

June 2012

The Nuffield Council on Bioethics publishes a report, *Novel techniques for the prevention of mitochondrial DNA disorders*.

The Human Fertilisation and Embryology Authority launches a public consultation exploring mitochondrial donation.

July 2012

The Human Fertilisation and Embryology Authority runs a series of public dialogue events across the UK.

March 2013

The Human Fertilisation and Embryology Authority publishes a report on their public consultation and updated scientific review, which concludes that mitochondrial donation techniques have potential to be used if safety and efficacy are refined, and that the public are broadly supportive.

June 2013

The Department of Health and the Human Fertilisation and Embryology Authority state that draft regulations to permit mitochondrial donation will be issued later in 2013, then taken to further public consultation.

March 2014

The Department of Health publishes draft regulations for mitochondrial donation. A public consultation is launched for three months.

The House of Commons holds an adjournment debate.

April 2014

A favourable evaluation of the Human Fertilisation and Embryology Authority's public dialogue and consultation is published.

June 2014

The Human Fertilisation and Embryology Authority releases its third scientific review of the safety and efficacy of mitochondrial donation. It reports that there is no evidence to suggest either technique is unsafe and both have potential to be used to prevent serious mitochondrial disease.

July 2014

The Department of Health publishes the Government's response to the public consultation on draft mitochondrial donation regulations.

September 2014

The House of Commons holds a backbenchers debate on mitochondrial donation.

December 2014

The Government publishes the Human Fertilisation and Embryology (Mitochondrial Donation) Regulations 2015.

January–February 2015

In the House of Lords peers vote by 280 to 48 (opens in a new tab) in support of the Human Fertilisation and Embryology (Mitochondrial Donation) Regulations 2015.

In the House of Commons MPs vote by 382 to 128 to pass the Human Fertilisation and Embryology (Mitochondrial Donation) Regulations 2015.

October 2015

The Human Fertilisation and Embryology (Mitochondrial Donation) Regulations 2015 come into effect.

The Human Fertilisation and Embryology Authority publishes provisions for licensing mitochondrial donation.

June 2016

Published in the journal *Nature*, scientists at the Wellcome Centre for Mitochondrial Research report the first in-depth analysis of human embryos created using a new technique designed to reduce the risk of mothers passing on mitochondrial disease to their children.

July 2016

Scientists at the Wellcome Centre for Mitochondrial Research develop a new genetic test for mitochondrial disease which can provide results in two to three days.

November 2016

An independent expert panel convened by the Human Fertilisation and Embryology Authority to undertake a review of mitochondrial donation techniques, recommends cautious adoption of the techniques in the clinic.

December 2016

The Human Fertilisation and Embryology Authority agree that clinics can now apply for a licence to carry out mitochondrial donation treatment.

March 2017

Researchers in Newcastle are given the first UK licence to carry out mitochondrial donation treatment.

⇨ The above information is reprinted with kind permission from the Wellcome Trust. Please visit www.wellcome.ac.uk for further information.

© Wellcome Trust 2017

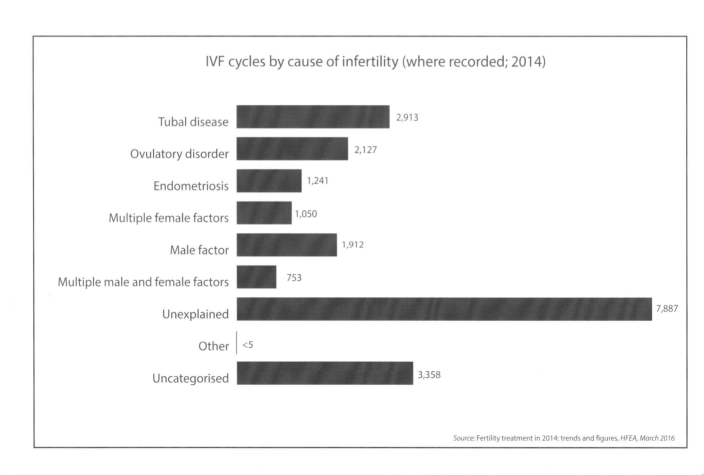

IVF cycles by cause of infertility (where recorded; 2014)

Tubal disease	2,913
Ovulatory disorder	2,127
Endometriosis	1,241
Multiple female factors	1,050
Male factor	1,912
Multiple male and female factors	753
Unexplained	7,887
Other	<5
Uncategorised	3,358

Source: Fertility treatment in 2014: trends and figures, HFEA, March 2016

A look inside the Czech Republic's booming fertility holiday industry

THE CONVERSATION

An article from **The Conversation.**

By Amy Speier, Assistant Professor of Anthropology, University of Texas Arlington

In 2008, a friend sent me a link to a Czech company called IVF Holiday. Clicking the link, I saw images of quaint European towns. These were accompanied by pictures of smiling white babies – and promises of affordable and safe rounds of in vitro fertilization (IVF).

I soon realized I'd stumbled into a new type of tourism: fertility holidays.

As a medical anthropologist, I knew I had to pursue this topic. Here was a perfect example of patients turning to medicine's global marketplace when high prices of health care back home block access to treatments.

I subsequently conducted three years of fieldwork in the Czech Republic and North America to trace the fertility journeys of 29 American reproductive tourists. Their stories are in my forthcoming book Fertility Holidays: IVF Tourism and the Reproduction of Whiteness.

A souvenir of a different sort

IVF is an assisted reproductive technology that increases the chances of conception for women or couples suffering from infertility. It monitors and stimulates a woman's ovulation, retrieves a woman's eggs and fertilizes the eggs with sperm in a lab. The fertilized egg or eggs are then transferred back to a woman's uterus. For women who suffer age-related infertility, they may need IVF using an egg donor.

However, costs in the United States for IVF can quickly become prohibitively expensive, running in the tens of thousands of dollars.

After looking further into IVF Holiday, I soon learned that it was owned by a married couple named Tom and Hana. Hana, a Czech woman, and Tom, an American from Ohio, learned early in their marriage that they would need IVF. With costs running as high as US$30,000, it was a procedure they simply couldn't afford in North America.

However, there was a cheaper option: in 1995, in order to counteract a declining birth rate, the Czech government had decided to insure women for three cycles of IVF.

In January 2006, Hana and Tom embarked for Hana's Moravian hometown and visited a clinic in Zlín. Pictures of their twins hugging one another show they returned home with the souvenir they sought.

Soon, the idea dawned on Hana and Tom to start a company that would help other lower-middle-class Americans travel to the Czech Republic to undergo IVF at a much lower cost. They realized they could act as intermediaries, providing transportation, travel recommendations and translators for all clinic visits.

IVF Holiday was born.

The typical fertility traveller

With companies like IVF Holiday paving the way, reproductive travel has become an increasingly popular option for North Americans who can't afford treatment in the U.S., but still long for babies of their own.

When many first encountered IVF Holiday's website, they felt empowered by the amount of information available. They spoke of reading endless online testimonials and contacting previous fertility tourists, acting as diligent consumers before making the decision to travel abroad for treatment.

Kay, a lawyer from the Northeast, travelled to the Zlín clinic in 2006 as one of the first North American patient clients seeking IVF.

When I interviewed her, she laughed as she recalled her first impression of the clinic – its large, rickety elevator that she took to the second floor of a former Communist-era building. Fearful of the elevator, she hesitated. Hana encouraged her to take this literal and metaphorical step. Thankfully, the door opened to the clinic that was the same clinic she'd seen on the IVF Holiday website.

So far, the North Americans travelling to the Czech Republic from North America have been predominantly white and lower- to middle-class. (I did interview one Puerto Rican couple and one African-American couple.) They're typically in their late 30's and early 40's, and their age-related infertility often means they need IVF using an egg donor.

The majority were well-versed in the world of assisted reproductive technologies (ARTs), having undergone several IUIs (intrauterine insemination) in the U.S., often with the help of fertility drugs. They may have even tried one or more IVF cycles, but couldn't continue due to financial constraints. North American reproductive tourists were also relatively well-travelled, although some were venturing abroad for the first time.

A number would end up staying at a small bed-and-breakfast in the hills of the town. This quaint bed-and-breakfast became a communal space for IVF travellers, many of whom became immediate friends, bonding over the fact they were undergoing IVF in a foreign country.

Contrasting costs

Back in the U.S., the reproductive medical industry is largely unregulated, and many have been critical of the commercial nature of a "baby business" that is largely profit-driven. Currently, there is no limit to the amount an egg donor can be paid – a number that typically ranges from $8,000 to $10,000. Given patient demand for reproductive technologies – and high profit margins – there's little incentive for clinics to reduce their prices.

Meanwhile, the Czech reproductive medical industry is also profiting. But it's from a lower price structure and liberal legislation that stipulates that sperm and egg donation must be voluntary and anonymous. While donors cannot be paid for their eggs, they're offered attractive compensatory payments of approximately 1,000 euros for the discomfort involved in ovarian stimulation and egg retrieval from the clinic. (This amounts to roughly three months' salary for egg donors.)

For North American patients travelling to the Czech Republic, treatment for IVF was $3,000. For an egg donor cycle, the cost was $4,000. On average, North Americans spent $10,000 for the entire trip. By comparison, a round of IVF with egg donation in the United States costs between $25,000 and $40,000.

A shifting business model

While IVF brokers were initially needed to facilitate travel between North America and the Czech Republic, their role has diminished significantly over the past decade.

Doctors were finding themselves answering too many direct questions through Hana, so in March 2009, the Zlín clinic hired its own coordinators. Previously, patients had to work with IVF Holiday as an intermediary; now they can work directly with the Czech clinic, which has become savvy at offering patient-centered care.

One of the new coordinator hires was a Czech woman named Lenka. The wife of a doctor who also works at the clinic, Lenka is a petite Slovak who has travelled extensively throughout the United States. As someone who also needed in vitro fertilization for her second child, she's able to empathize with the pain of infertility. Like Hana, she's able to deftly bridge Czech and American cultural differences.

In 2010, Lenka had been the only coordinator at the Zlín clinic. But when I visited the summer of 2014, I was struck by the cramped quarters of a larger office, where there were eight cubicles facing one another – and eight women typing emails or on the phone speaking Russian, Italian, French and English. Furthermore, the clinic built its own en suite accommodations for foreign patients, cutting the favoured bed-and-breakfast out of the profits.

I quickly discovered that North American patients had become a very small piece of the Czech reproductive tourism pie. In a clinic in Prague, there's a world map

in the main conference center with the heading Nase Deti v Svete: Our Children in the World. You can see pins in every country where a recipient couple had IVF using egg donor in the Czech Republic. wwwClinics are also opening farther east, in countries like Hungary and the Ukraine. While this may detract from the profits of Czech clinics, with more and more international consumers becoming aware of fertility tourism's viability and affordability, it's a market that's ripe for growth.

17 March 2016

⇨ The above information is reprinted with kind permission from *The Conversation*. Please visit www. theconversation.com for further information.

Abortion guidance ignores gender complexity, says BMA

New government guidance on abortion fails to address the complexities and legalities around gender, the BMA has warned.

The Department of Health produced updated rules after the CPS (Crown Prosecution Service) highlighted a lack of guidance on abortion law as a problem area for doctors.

Guidance in Relation to Requirements of the Abortion Act 1967 states that abortion on the grounds of gender is not lawful.

It adds that the two doctors required to approve abortions must consider women's individual circumstances and be ready to justify decisions. This is in response to concerns about the use of pre-signed forms.

BMA ethics committee chair Tony Calland said that, while overall the new guidance contained helpful clarification of issues concerning abortion law, the association had some concerns about it.

Exceptional circumstances

Dr Calland said: "We feel that it fails to reflect the complexities and full legal situation regarding abortion and gender."

He said while the BMA believes it is "normally unethical" to terminate a pregnancy on the basis of foetal sex, there could be exceptional circumstances not covered in the guidance.

"We recognise that in some cases doctors may come to the conclusion that the effects of having a child of a particular gender are so severe to the physical or mental health of the pregnant woman as to provide legal and ethical justification for an abortion," he said. "This is in addition to the gender-related serious foetal abnormalities referred to in the DH's guidance."

In August 2013, the CPS highlighted the lack of guidance when explaining its decision not to prosecute two doctors for certifying abortions based on the gender of the foetus.

It said: "There is no guidance on how a doctor should go about assessing the risk to physical or mental health, no guidance on where the threshold of risk lies and no guidance on a proper process for recording the assessment carried out."

The new guidance does not change the law in relation to abortion, but is intended to provide support for doctors by setting out how the law is interpreted by the Department of Health.

30 June 2016

⇨ The above information is reprinted with kind permission from the British Medical Association. Please visit www.bma.org.uk for further information.

New parents in the UK admit to feeling 'gender disappointment' if their child is the 'wrong' sex

"It's worth remembering a child isn't their gender."

A quarter of mums in the UK admit to feeling "very disappointed" if their child is the "wrong" sex - ie. not the sex they'd hoped for.

A further 3% said this affected their ability to bond with their child long term and 6% would consider flying abroad for gender selection IVF, which is currently illegal in the UK.

Mothers are twice as likely to want daughters over sons, the survey of 2,189 UK mums from parenting site ChannelMum.com found. While dads are three times more likely to want a baby boy.

ChannelMum's founder, Siobhan Freegard, believes it is important this feeling is spoken about openly, but adds that understanding a child is not defined by their sex can help new parents to overcome this feeling of disappointment.

"Boy or girl – every child is a blessing, but the issue of gender disappointment is something we need to talk about and bring into the open," said Freegard.

"With mums and dads often at odds about the gender they really want, one parent will usually end up disappointed, so we must ensure families have the support they need to bond with their baby," Freegard continued.

"It's worth remembering a child isn't their gender – they are their own people with their own personality. So whatever the gender, let your child be who they are, not what you hoped them to be."

The majority (80%) of mums questioned said they believe it's normal to have a preference on the gender of your child.

Yasmeen Hassan, Equality Now's global executive director and mum of two boys, told The Huffington Post UK that she can relate, as she herself had a preference for girls.

"As a women's rights activist I always thought I wanted two children and they would be girls – as I have so much to share with, and teach, a girl," she said.

"Before my sons were born I didn't think the same would be possible with boys. But after having the boys I figured out that it is actually a great privilege to be a strong mother of boys, because you can bring up feminist boys."

Hassan added that she can't relate to the feeling of disappointment linked to gender preference.

"My experience was I had these children and immediately they were individuals," she explained.

"I looked at them from the time they were born and they had very distinct personalities and I realised it is such an honour to know this person and to explore who they are and what they will become.

"It seems to me that the disappointment comes when people have a vision of what different-gendered children can do. For instance, if they've always imagined playing baseball with their child and they believe that child has to be a boy for that dream to be possible.

"The disappointment may also arise if they want to see their child as an extension of themselves. I've seen some parents who say, 'I didn't get to do this, so my son will get to do x, y and z,' and if they don't have that son then there's a disappointment.

"So to avoid disappointment you have to stop looking at children as an extension of yourself or as a gender stereotype. Instead, see them as individuals who can be anything that they want."

The study also revealed the most common reasons parents gave for wanting a child of a certain sex. Top reason for wanting girls included: girls stay closer to their parents when they grow up (41%); girls are more fun to dress up (40%); and girls are better behaved (7%).

While the top reasons for wanting boys were: boys are easier (14%); boys are more fun to play with (9%); or cultural reasons (4%).

Dr Tamara Kayali Browne, lecturer in health ethics and professionalism at Deakin University, Australia, recently wrote about sex selection in a blog on *The Guardian*'s Comment Is Free.

She explained that parents hoping to get a specific parenting experience based on their child's sex may be denying themselves and their children a fulfilling relationship.

"According to the state of the evidence so far, there is no biological reason why parents can't have the sort of bond and experiences they want with a child of any sex," she wrote.

"Despite more than 100 years of research, scientific studies have failed to provide good evidence to support the belief that babies are born with something like a 'male brain' or a 'female brain' which causes the gender traits parents have in mind.

"If you play dolls with your son or football with your daughter, their brains will not explode."

21 April 2017

⇨ The above information is reprinted with kind permission from The Huffington Post UK. Please visit www.huffingtonpost.co.uk for further information.

© 2017 AOL (UK) Limited

Three-parent children

The background

In 2008 Parliament passed a law that gave the Government the power to introduce regulations allowing three-parent embryos. The Government made an assurance that regulations would only be considered once it was clear that the scientific procedures were safe.

The Government asked the Human Fertilisation and Embryology Authority (HFEA) to assess the safety and effectiveness of the procedure. The HFEA concluded that evidence did not indicate that the techniques are unsafe although it accepted that there was little evidence due to the fact that such procedures are so novel. The HFEA suggested that additional research be carried out to provide further safety information.

Last year the Government gave its support to the technique, after the HFEA said that a consultation on three-parent embryos was broadly supported by the public. If Parliament approves of the regulations then the first three-parent baby could be born in Britain by 2015.

The science

Supporters of the technique claim that it could eliminate mitochondrial disease, a genetic condition passed from mother to child. Mitochondria are the tiny, biological 'power stations' found in human cells that give the body energy. Defects in the mitochondria can cause a range of serious problems including muscular dystrophy. On average, one child in 6,500 is affected by a serious mitochondrial disease which may, in some instances, lead to death in infancy.

The technique involves collecting eggs from a mother with damaged mitochondria and a donor with healthy mitochondria. Doctors would then destroy the nucleus of the donor's egg and insert the mother's nucleus in its place. The donor's egg with the mother's nucleus now in it would then be fertilised by the father.

The concerns

(1) Safety

Supporters of the techniques have no way of predicting what the long-term consequences will be. Furthermore, the risks involved in this process are not limited to the first generation; all future generations will be subject to risk. The procedures involve cell nuclear replacement which has not yet been shown to work in humans. Whilst it appears to be effective in lower mammals like mice, use of such techniques in higher mammals has led to a considerable number of miscarriages and the birth of large numbers of abnormal offspring. The Food and Drug Administration agency (FDA) in the United States has warned that there is not enough data in animals or in humans to move on to these new techniques. The HFEA are clearly concerned about the effects such techniques could have on future generations and have advised that children born from these techniques should be monitored for a long period of time after birth. In March 2014, the Government asked the HFEA to conduct a third safety review of the techniques. It is clear that the Government should have waited for a conclusion before drafting the regulations.

(2) Identity of the future child

These new procedures have significant implications for the understanding of human life. More than two individuals are participating in the generation of new life and therefore more than two people must be considered as parents. Moreover, the genes from the third person will be passed on down the generations and will be impossible to remove from the family. This raises serious issues of personal and family identity for children born as a result of these techniques.

(3) Engineering the genes of future generations

The intention of these new techniques is to alter the genes passed on to the new generation. This is ethically controversial, as no future generation will have given their consent to the procedures. No country in the world makes provision for such developments. The World Health Organization has said, "germ-cell therapy, where there is an intention or possibility of altering the genes passed on to the next generation, should not be permitted in the foreseeable future. The Council of Europe's Convention on Human Rights and Biomedicine explicitly prohibits these measures.

(4) A new eugenics?

This would be the first time intentional genetic alterations of descendants are considered and may give rise to further genetic alterations of human beings. Professor Lord Robert Winston has warned that major advances in genetic technologies could lead to a form of child "eugenics" that could have serious implications for the individuals involved and society in general. He says "we may find that people will want to modify their children, enhance their intelligence, their strength and their beauty and all the other so-called desirable characteristics. 13 doctors and professors in the field of genetics or bioethics wrote to *The Guardian* newspaper warning them that the move "risks dehumanising and commodifying relationships between children and their parents."

CARE's response

The current developments in the UK are unprecedented and are prohibited in almost every other Western country for good public safety and ethical reasons. In light of the ethical arguments relating to the undermining of the sense of identity of future generations, intrusion of a third party into the reproductive exclusivity of a couple, the biological risk to future generations and the legitimate fears about the long-term consequences of altering genes, it is clear that we should not be going down this route. Instead we should be focusing on finding real treatments for people suffering from mitochondrial disease and better support for them and their families. Further, Christians must continue to proclaim the inherent value of all life, regardless of its state of health.

⇨ The above information is reprinted with kind permission from CARE. Please visit www.care.org.uk for further information.

© Care 2017

'Three-parent baby' born: world's first child with two biological mothers and one biological father

The baby boy was conceived using a controversial technique.

By Ellen Wallwork

A 'three-parent baby' has been born, in a world first for reproductive science.

The five-month-old boy is genetically related to two women and one man.

He was conceived using a controversial technique that incorporates DNA from three people, which was developed with the aim of eliminating inherited diseases.

"To save lives is the ethical thing to do," embryologist Dr John Zhang, told *The New Statesman*.

Abrahim's Jordanian parents were treated by a US-based team in Mexico.

His mother carries the gene mutation for Leigh syndrome, a progressive disorder that affects the central nervous system and which killed her first two children.

She carries the mutation in about a quarter of her mitochondria (which provide energy for our cells).

The mother and her husband sought the help of Dr Zhang, medical director at the New Hope Fertility Center in New York City, US.

The couple's son was conceived using an approach called spindle nuclear transfer. The nucleus from one of the mother's eggs was inserted into an egg from an anonymous donor, which was fertilised using the father's sperm.

Five embryos were created, only one of which developed normally and was implanted in the mother's womb.

While the US has not approved the technique, Mexico has "no rules", Dr Zhang is reported to have said.

Tests of the baby's mitochondria showed that less than 1% carried the Leigh mutation, which is thought to be too low a level to cause any problems.

Last year the House of Lords approved legislation to allow a different form of "three-parent technique" called mitochondrial transfer, making the UK the first country in the world explicitly to approve the procedure.

Mitochondrial transfer involves fertilising both the mother's egg and a donor egg with the father's sperm. The eggs' nuclei are removed before the fertilised eggs start dividing into early stage embryos. The nucleus from the donor's fertilised egg is discarded and replaced by that from the mother's fertilised egg.

Strict controls remain in force in the UK and scientists wishing to employ the technique would first have to obtain permission from the Human Fertilisation and Embryology Authority.

Professor Doug Turnbull, from the University of Newcastle, told the Press Association: "There have been extensive discussions in the UK to ensure that families with mitochondrial disease get the best possible advice about their reproductive options and that any new IVF-based technique is appropriately regulated and funded.

"This abstract gives very little information about the technique used, the follow-up of the child or the ethical approval process."

28 September 2016

⇨ The above information is reprinted with kind permission from The Huffington Post UK. Please visit www.huffingtonpost.co.uk for further information.

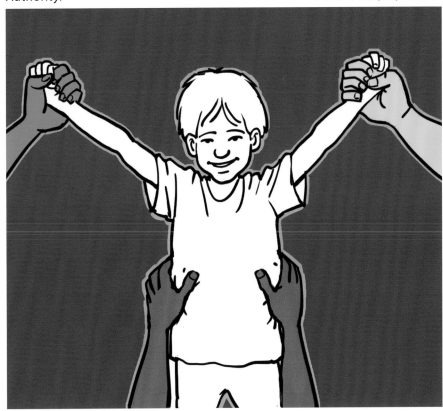

Key facts

- Women of childbearing age have a period approximately every 28 days, although the length of the cycle can vary and between 24 and 35 days is common. (page 1)

- An egg can be fertilised by sperm during the 12 to 24 hours after it has been released from the ovaries. (page 1)

- Around one in seven couples may have difficulty conceiving. This is approximately 3.5 million people in the UK. (page 2)

- About 84% of couples will conceive naturally within one year if they have regular unprotected sex (every two or three days). (page 2)

- For couples who've been trying to conceive for more than three years without success, the likelihood of getting pregnant naturally within the next year is 25% or less. (page 2)

- According to the NHS, approximately one third of fertility problems are due to issues with the female, one third are down to problems with the male, and in up to 23% of circumstances doctors are unable to pinpoint a cause. (page 3)

- Around 80% of both sexes believe women's fertility only starts to decline after the age of 35, and a quarter of boys think women's fertility starts to decline after the age of 40, compared with 16% of girls. Two-thirds of those surveyed think men's fertility only starts declining after the age of 40, with a third believing it doesn't begin declining until after the age of 50. While the change is less dramatic for men, fertility rates for both sexes actually decline gradually from the late 20s, and can be affected by genetic and environmental factors such as smoking, obesity and nutrition. (page 5)

- The vast majority of young people – around nine in ten – are aware that women are most fertile under the age of 30. (page 6)

- Encouragingly, 80% of girls and two-thirds of boys (66%) are aware that age is the number one factor which affects female fertility. (page 6)

- 40% of girls mistakenly believe that having a miscarriage or being on the contraceptive pill for too long can adversely affect fertility. (page 6)

- just over half (53%) of younger women diagnosed with breast cancer have no discussion with healthcare professionals about fertility preservation options, including freezing embryos or eggs, according to new findings from Breast Cancer Care. (page 8)

- The majority (86%) of almost 500 younger women surveyed by Breast Cancer Care said they received chemotherapy, a treatment that can cause infertility. The survey also revealed more than a quarter (28%) of younger women with breast cancer would like to have a child or add to their family after treatment. (page 8)

- In more than 40% of cases where couples struggle to conceive, the underlying fertility issue is linked to sperm abnormalities. (page 9)

- Currently just over 25% of all IVF cycles result in a live birth. This naturally varies woman to woman, and a fertility specialist will be able to give a more accurate and personalised likelihood of success. It is important to be realistic but positive about the chances of success. (page 21)

- From a survey of all women who started IVF and intracytoplasmic sperm injection (ICSI) in the UK from 1999 to 2008 using their own eggs and partner's sperm (114,000 women who completed almost 185,000 cycles of treatment) 29.1% had a live birth following their first cycle. And 43% had a baby following six cycles of treatment. (page 22)

- By 54% to 26%, the British public support making it legal to pay a surrogate. (page 28)

- Approximately one in 200 children in the UK are born with faulty mitochondrial DNA. While many people have mild or no symptoms, around one in 6,500 may develop more serious mitochondrial disorders. (page 33)

- For North American patients travelling to the Czech Republic, treatment for IVF was $3,000. For an egg donor cycle, the cost was $4,000. On average, North Americans spent $10,000 for the entire trip. By comparison, a round of IVF with egg donation in the United States costs between $25,000 and $40,000. (page 36)

- An estimated 20,000 IVF cycles were completed in the Czech Republic in 2006, a quarter of which were for foreign couples. By 2014, that number had grown to 30,000, with foreign couples accounting for one-third of the total. (page 36)

- A quarter of mums in the UK admit to feeling "very disappointed" if their child is the "wrong" sex - ie. not the sex they'd hoped for. (page 37)

- The majority (80%) of mums questioned said they believe it's normal to have a preference on the gender of your child. (page 37)

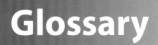
Adoption

When a family becomes the legal guardians (adoptive parents) for a child who cannot be brought up by his or her biological parents. Couples who are infertile but wish to have a child look to adoption as an alternative. More recently, laws regarding adoption from overseas have become less strict.

ART/Artificial Reproductive Technology

'Fertility treatments': achieving pregnancy through artificial means.

Designer baby

A term coined by journalists, this refers to the use of gene therapy to determine what a baby will look like. There is a fear that this will lead to people using technology to select and 'customise' their baby before it's even born – selecting sex, height, appearance, eye/hair colour and possibly even IQ.

Donor/Donor rights

A donor is someone who donates either their eggs (female) or sperm (male) to be used in fertility treatments to help people who are unable to have children of their own. Donors used to remain completely anonymous, but in 2005 the law changed so that when donor-conceived children reach 18, they can find out the identity of the donor and whether they have any half-brothers or sisters (though this largely depends on whether they are ever told they are donor-conceived).

Eugenics

The belief that the human population can be improved through controlled breeding to increase the likelihood of more desirable heritable characteristics. For example, the Nazi party believed the Aryan race to be a master race and therefore their blonde hair and blue eyes were seen as superior characteristics.

Fertility/Infertility

According to doctors, infertility is when a couple are unable to become pregnant despite having regular, unprotected, sex for two years. There are a number of possible reasons for couples to be infertile. For example, male's low sperm count, damage to a female's fallopian tubes, etc.

Genetic testing

This refers to a technique called pre-implantation genetic diagnosis (PGD). This allows parents to test for serious genetically inherited conditions such Huntington's disease or cystic fibrosis. There is a fear that genetic testing will be misused (see *Designer baby*). However, it can be legally carried out if it is in the best interest for the embryo.

IVF (In vitro fertilisation)

IVF literally means 'fertilisation in glass', giving us the familiar term 'test tube baby'. IVF treatment is considered by couples who are having fertility problems and are not getting pregnant. Eggs are removed from the ovaries and fertilised with sperm in a laboratory dish before being placed in the woman's womb.

Saviour sibling

A child who is conceived because they will be a guaranteed tissue match for their sibling, who is affected with a fatal disease. Blood is collected from the saviour sibling's umbilical cord and can then be used to treat their unwell brother or sister. This is a very controversial procedure as some people feel it is wrong to conceive a child with the sole purpose of saving another. The procedure is only permitted if there are no matching tissue donors available anywhere else.

Surrogacy

When a couple who are unable to conceive naturally find another woman, known as the surrogate, to carry and give birth to their baby. Surrogacy is legal in the UK, but it is illegal to pay for the service. It is legal, however, to pay towards reasonable expenses such as medical costs.

Three-parent IVF

The process of creating a baby with three sets of DNA, rather than just the two – from the mother and father. This technique intends to help prevent inherited disorders as scientists can remove unhealthy mitochondria and replace them with healthy ones from a donor.

Assignments

Brainstorming

⇨ In small groups, discuss what you know about fertility.

- What is IVF?

- What age is a person most fertile?

- What kinds of things can affect a person's fertility?

Research

⇨ Choose a country outside of the EU and investigate is laws surrounding fertility treatment, surrogacy and adoption. Write a short essay, summarising your findings.

⇨ Research the different causes of infertility, in both men and women, and make a bullet point list. Share your findings with your class.

⇨ Conduct a survey throughout your year group to find out how many young people have thought about their fertility and considered whether they will want children in the future. Ask at least three different questions and create a series of graphs to demonstrate your findings.

⇨ Research fostering and adoption agencies in your area and create a leaflet for anyone who might be considering either of these options, explaining the first steps they should take and the potential benefits.

Design

⇨ Age is an important factor when it comes to fertility and a lot of women do not realise they have a problem until they try to conceive. Create a campaign that will raise awareness of the things that younger women can do to protect their fertility. Your campaign could take the form of posters, television adverts or leaflets, but try to consider which one of these would appeal most to a younger demographic.

⇨ Design a leaflet that explains the risks and benefits of IVF treatment.

⇨ Imagine there is a website called 'Surrogates R Us' where surrogate mothers and prospective parents can create profiles and contact one another. With a partner, design a prospective parent's profile. Your profile should include some personal information such as occupation, location, hobbies and beliefs. It should also include an advert specifying what you would like your surrogate to be like.

⇨ To take this further, consider whether you think it should be legal in the UK to advertise for surrogates/parents and create a bullet point list of pros and cons.

⇨ Design a questionnaire that will investigate opinions surrounding IVF for same-sex couples. Try to distribute your questionnaire across a range of sexes and age-groups. Analyse your results and write a summary, including graphs.

Oral

⇨ With a partner, discuss the emotional and physical effects that IVF can have on couples. Consider both female and the male perspective. Make some notes and feedback to your class.

⇨ Choose an illustration from this book and, in pairs, discuss what you think the artist was trying to portray with this image. Does the illustration work well with its accompanying article? If not, why not? How would you change it?

⇨ Mr and Mrs Turner both carry the gene for a genetic condition know as Sanfilippo syndrome. There is no cure for this disorder. They want to use IVF to select a healthy embryo and guarantee they have a child without Sanfilippo syndrome. In pairs, discuss the moral issues that are raised by this situation. Feedback and compare notes with the rest of your class.

⇨ Create a PowerPoint presentation that will explain the issue of fertility to young people and highlight some things they should do to safeguard their fertility for the future.

Reading/writing

⇨ Write a blog voicing your opinion about IVF treatment for women who are over the age of 40. Do you think treatment should be funded by the NHS? Do you think there should be a cut-off-age at which IVF is not permitted? Maybe you think it's okay, as long as the woman is paying to have the treatment privately?

⇨ Watch the film *My Sister's Keeper* (2009), or read the book of the same title by Jodi Picoult. Choose a character from the film/book and write a diary entry from their point of view, exploring their emotions and thoughts towards the concept of 'saviour siblings'.

⇨ Sex selection is a controversial issue. Write a newspaper column in which you strongly agree or disagree with the process of sex selection. You should back-up your argument with further research such as statistics and facts.

⇨ Read the article on page 37 and think of what you could say to someone who has admitted they were disappointed when they discovered the gender of their baby. Write an email, assuming you are this person's friend.